"Comprehensive"

Very few books about brain injury, if any, are as comprehensive and far-reaching as Dr. Stoler's. *Coping With Mild Traumatic Brain Injury* answers many questions haunting survivors and family members. I strongly recommend this text as required reading for anyone affiliated with the brain injury community.

George A. Zitnay, Ph.D.
President and CEO, Brain Injury Association

"Remarkable"

Diane Stoler has written a remarkable book. Her description of the neurologic, emotional, and psychological consequences of traumatic brain injury is encyclopedic, and will be instructive not only to survivors and their families, but also to every professional who works in this field. At the same time, something else emerges in this text, and that is the indomitable strength of the human spirit.

Joseph Ratner, M.D.
Chief of Psychiatry, HealthSouth/New England Rehabilitation Hospital

"Thorough and Practical"

Coping With Mild Traumatic Brain Injury is a thorough, practical guide through unfamiliar and often frightening territory, offering wisdom and hope.

Sally Jessy Raphael
Talk Show Host and Mother of a Person Who Sustained an MTBI

"A Must"

This book is a must-read for anyone who has experienced a mild brain injury, as well as for family members, friends, and professionals working in this area of treatment. In addition to providing valuable knowledge, it provides hope and inspiration for the future, from someone who has been there. It is the first book available for the many people who struggle with the "unseen injury"providing for them a reference guide to follow during their treatment and recovery.

Pat Lazarek
Resource Coordinator, Massachusetts Brain Injury Association

Coping
with Mild
Traumatic
Brain
Injury

Diane Roberts Stoler, EdD
Barbara Albers Hill

Avery Publishing Group
Garden City Park, New York

This book includes medical information and advice. The contents are current and accurate; however, the information presented is not intended to substitute for professional medical advice. We strongly urge you to consult with your physician or other qualified health-care provider prior to starting any new treatment, or if you have any questions regarding a medical condition.

The excerpt on page 249 is from "From Inside Out" by Beverley Bryant, which appeared in Through This Window: Views on Traumatic Brain Injury, edited by Patricia Felton, published by EBTS, Inc., 1992. Reprinted by permission.

Cover design: William Gonzalez and Rudy Shur
Original illustrations: William Gonzalez
In-house editor: Amy C. Tecklenburg
Typesetter: Al Berotti and Elaine V. McCaw
Printer: Paragon Press, Honesdale, PA

Avery Publishing Group, Inc.
120 Old Broadway
Garden City Park, NY 11040
1-800-548-5757

Library of Congress Cataloging-in-Publication Data

Stoler, Diane.
    Coping with mild traumatic brain injury : a guide to living with
the problems associated with brain trauma / Diane Stoler, Barbara
Albers Hill.
        p. cm.
    Includes bibliographical references and index.
    ISBN 0-89529-791-4
    1. Brain damage. 2. Brain—Wounds and injuries—Complications.
3. Brain damage—Patients—Rehabilitation. 4. Brain damage—
Psychological aspects.   I. Hill, Barbara Albers. II. Title.
RC387.5.S75 1998
616.8—dc21
                                                                    97-36528
                                                                        CIP

Printed in the United States of America

10 9 8 7 6 5 4 3 2 1

CONTENTS

To all people who have experienced a brain injury:
The human spirit is stronger than anything that can happen to it.
If there is a will, there is a way.

ACKNOWLEDGMENTS

This book is the result of countless hours of research along with a great number of experts in various fields who freely gave their time and commitment to its success. Each chapter was reviewed several times for accuracy of information. With deep gratitude, I want to thank the following experts for their contributions in specific subject areas:

For neurology, Jorge A. Gonzalez, M.D., A.B.P.N., Co-Medical Director, HealthSouth Rehabilitation Hospital, Tulsa, Oklahoma; Edward Bromfield, M.D., A.B.P.N., Assistant Professor of Neurology, Harvard Medical School, and Director, EEG Lab and Epilepsy Program, Brigham & Women's Hospital, Boston, Massachusetts; Linda Cowell, M.D., F.A.B.P.N., of Spaulding Rehabilitation Hospital; and April Mott, M.D., A.B.I.N., Assistant Professor, Department of Medicine, University of Connecticut Health Center, Taste and Smell Center, Farmington, Connecticut.

For neuropsychology, Barbara Bruno-Golden, Ed.D., a clinical neuropsychologist in private practice in Newton, Massachusetts.

For psychopharmacology, Jeffrey Hoffman, M.D., A.B.P.N., and Albert Koegler, M.D., A.B.P.N, psychopharmacologists in private practice in Lynnfield and Danvers, Massachusetts, respectively.

For psychology, Jack Jordon, Ph.D., Director, Family Loss Project/Network, Sherborn, Massachusetts, and Alma Dell Smith, Ph.D., A.B.P.P., Assistant Clinical Professor of Medicine (Psychology), Boston University Medical School.

For psychiatric nursing Ann Kennedy, M.S.N., R.N., Instructor, Northeastern University, Boston, Massachusetts.

For internal medicine, Susan Beluk, M.D., F.A.B.P., of Spaulding Rehabilitation Hospital, Boston.

For ophthalmology, Dennis F. Stoler, M.D., F.A.C.O., of Microsurgical Eye Associates, Danvers, Massachusetts.

For otolaryngology, Terry J. Garfinkle, M.D., F.A.C.S., Assistant Professor, Harvard Medical School, and Pediatric Instructor, Tufts University School of Medicine, Boston, Massachusetts; and James L. Demetroulakos, M.D., F.A.C.S., Assistant Professor, Harvard Medical School, and Pediatric Instructor, Tufts University School of Medicine, Boston, Massachusetts.

For orthopedics, Kenneth Glazier, M.D., an orthopedist in private practice in Newburyport, Massachusetts.

For physiatry, Paul Corcorian, M.D., of Spaulding Rehabilitation Hospital, Boston, Massachusetts, and Lecturer, Harvard Medical School.

For rehabilitation, Karen Lucas, Ph.D., C.C.C.-S.L.P., Director of Rehabilitation Services, Greenery Extended Care, Danvers, Massachusetts; Elise Paquette R.N., C.R.R., Program Consultant and former Inpatient Program Director, Northeast Rehabilitation Hospital, Salem, New Hampshire; and Judy Romano, OT-R, Occupational Therapy Team Leader/Outpatient Services, HealthSouth/New England Rehabilitation Hospital, Woburn, Massachusetts.

For treatment approaches, Igor Burdenko, Ph.D., Director, Burdenko Institute, Lexington, Massachusetts (the Burdenko method); Nancy Risley, R.P.P., President/Director, and Kris Stecker, R.P.P., Director, Polarity Realization Institute, Ipswitch, Massachusetts (polarity therapy); Juliet McCoy-Needham, a Feldenkrais practitioner in private practice in North Andover, Massachusetts (Feldenkrais method); David Sollars, Lic.Ac, a homeopath, herbalist, and acupuncturist in private practice in Northhampton, Massachusetts (homeopathics, herbs, and acupuncture); Paul Swingle, Ph.D., psychophysiologist and Instructor, Harvard Medical School (EEG biofeedback); Judy Smith, OT-R, of Spaulding Rehabilitation Hospital, Medford, Massachusetts (EMG biofeedback); Ken Spracklin, P.T., of North Andover Physical Therapy Associates, North Andover, Massachusetts (physical therapy); and Mark Delorenzo, D.C., Instructor, Palmer Chiropractic College, Davenport, Iowa, and a chiropractor in private practice in Andover, Massachusetts (chiropractic).

For information about specific symptom topics, Steve Labov, Member, Board of Governors, American Council for Headache Education, and Joan Clover, Co-Facilitator for ACHE/Prodigy, Headache Support (headaches); Darlene Herrick (sensory problems); and Ruth Ruderman, Speech and Language Pathologist, Lexington Public Schools, Lexington, Massachusetts (academic skills deficits).

For legal issues, Kenneth Kolpan, Esq., an attorney in private practice in Boston, Massachusetts, and Charles N. Simkins, Esq., Simkins & Simkins, Northville, Michigan.

For insurance issues, Nancy Burns and Janet Papineau at William J. Cleary Insurance, Boston.

For background and general information about traumatic brain injury, Mary Reitter, Program Director at the national headquarters of the Brain Injury Association, Washington, DC; Elizabeth Jenkins, Executive Director, and Beth Lundgren (Watusi), at the Brain Injury Association of Kansas and Greater Kansas City; Elaine M. Boucher, Executive Assistant, New Hampshire Brain Injury Association; and Pat Lazarek, Resource Coordinator, Mary Forde, Administrative Assistant and Events Coordinator, Rosalie Berquist, Prevention Coordinator, and Anne Marie Flavin, Administrative Assistant of the Prevention Program, with the Massachusetts Brain Injury Association.

In addition to all of the professionals named above, special thanks and appreciation go to the following people with mild traumatic brain injury, who all volunteered their time to proofread this book to insure that its contents related to the needs of brain-injured people: Gracia Berry, Elaine Boucher, Barbara Sweeny, and Pat Davis. Pat also helped to proofread the final copy. Her love and friendship throughout the project kept me focused and my spirits high. Thanks go also to Lisa Anastos, who had no previous knowledge of the topic and was willing to listen for clarity of information.

Deep appreciation goes to Fran Rand for her support, encouragement, and the many hours that she and my husband, Denny Stoler, spent in proofing the first several drafts of the book.

My deepest gratitude goes to the following people, who have allowed me to share their stories with you: Shari Aznoian-Wilson, Jack Bateman, Gracia Berry, Elaine Boucher, Beverley Bryant, John Carter, Sharron Carter, Mike Deloge, Patricia Felton, Mary Beth Farr, Lianne Hansen, Darlene Herrick, Diane Holmes, Robert Holmes, Kevin Hurley, Missy Kelly, Randi Kleinstein, Helen Kronenfeld, Morris Kronenfeld, Terrie McKenna, Deborah McLean, Laurel Perkins, Barbara Perry, Jackie Nink Pflug, Rita Smithuysen, Dena Taylor, Gail Willeke, and others, whose names do not appear because of ongoing litigation.

I am grateful to the supportive staff of Avery Publishing Group. Special thanks go to the late Roger Nye and to Rudy Shur, Joanne Abrams, Karen Hay, and Amy Tecklenburg, my editor, whose questions and calmness helped me to define the focus of this book. Very special thanks to my coauthor Barbara Albers Hill, whose help, guidance, and support were invaluable. And thanks to her husband, Kevin, and their three children, for sharing Barbara with me during this project.

Thanks also to the many professionals who helped me with my recovery, for without their help I truly doubt I could have written this book: Dr. Michael Scott, Dr. James Whitlock, Dr. Ed Bromfield, Lucille Leonard, Dr. Igor Burdenko, Dr. Paul Swingle, Judy Smith, Ken Spracklin, SusanJane Brewster, Lynn Mascato, Michelle Skane, Lisa Orcutt-Murphy, Beth Quintal, Dr. Mark Delorenzo, Jean Crannell,

Coping With Mild Traumatic Brain Injury

David Sollars, Sarah Eames, Maratha Rossman, Dominic Secondiani, Juliet McCoy-Needham, Betty Woodsum, and attorneys William Troupe, Carmine DiAdamo, and Ted Fairburn.

Special words of appreciation and love to the various people whose love, support, and understanding have helped my recovery. To my mentor and dear friend Eugene Isotti, Ph.D., thank you for your wisdom and for believing in me even when I did not. Thank you to Nancy Isotti, Jacqui Pilgrim, Fran Rand, David Rand, Barbara Bruno-Golden, Sharyn Russell, Ann Kennedy, Sandra and Jack Hawxwell, Joyce and Normal Spector, the late Amy Silberman, the late Kathi Savage, Julie Joseph, Karen Callahan, Kathy and Rick Murdock, Francine Kaplan, Judy Russo, Gale and Jimer Wood, Fran Iseman, Rose Ann Negele, Susan Glazier, Sandi Perchik, Lynn Koplowitz, Ellie DiCataldo, and Gail Willeke, for their friendship. To my many Prodigy TBI friends, such as Rita Smithuysen, Shirl Rapport, Sunny Sheila Underwood, Jeri Dopp, Samantha Jane Scolamiero, and Carollee Crabtree, and to many I have never met, for their prayers and support. To my extended family members, Helen and Morris Kronenfeld, Shirley and Joe Stoler, Elaine Rembrandt and Rabbi Daniel Roberts, Evette Mittin Horrow, Patti and Lee Schear, Cathy and Frank Ginocchi, Pegi Stoler, Phyllis Goodman, Irv and Roz Pocrass, Faye Ross, and Tippy and Erwin Awerbuch.

Lastly, my love and very special appreciation goes to my husband, Denny, and our three children, Craig, Brad, and Alan. They never lost faith in me and that I would recover. It was their continual love, support, and encouragement that kept my hope alive. Thank you for being there for me.

It must be evident that I have received valuable help and support from many directions. If I have forgotten to mention your name, please know that you yourself are not forgotten. I thank you.

FOREWORD

Until very recently, the emotional and cognitive consequences of brain injury were largely overlooked and unknown to many, including patients and those close to them. Even today, the profound changes that people experience following brain injury are often misinterpreted as signs of irresponsibility, a lack of motivation, neurotic behavior, or a litigation-prone personality. People with obviously disabling conditions stand a better chance of being recognized as needing medical care. Mild traumatic brain injury (MTBI) is more likely to be overlooked or its symptoms dismissed. The misdiagnosed patient is then very likely to experience a downward spiral of neglect, frustration, and economic loss, leading quite often to torment and despair. Spouse, family, employer, and coworkers alike may notice that the individual appears changed, but they can become frustrated when their well-meaning efforts to help are ineffective or only seem make matters worse. The disruption of a once-solid marriage and family is not uncommon, adding to the brain-injured person's mounting difficulties.

As doctors, we are aware of the need to give our patients as much information as possible. Unfortunately, all too often, we enter a patient's room with the intention of answering every possible question from the patient and his or her family only to have the pager beep unexpectedly or a diligent staff member track us down to inform us that our presence is urgently needed elsewhere. For years, clinicians in the field of traumatic brain injury have needed a way to provide comprehensive, useful information that would enable patients, family, and friends to gain a better understanding of the many events that can follow a head injury.

With this book, we finally have a way to bridge the knowledge gap between clinicians who routinely work with MTBI patients and people who are exposed to this condition for the first time. It is, in a sense, a beginner's manual to help the layperson understand what is involved in the diagnosis, treatment, and rehabilitation of brain-injured people, written by a person whom I greatly admire—a clinician who has firsthand experience of what it is like not only to treat this type of injury, but to endure and recover from it as well.

This book will serve to better educate people and help them to recognize that brain injury is a treatable condition that deserves greater awareness, and to understand that those who experience MTBI deserve appropriate attention and treatment.

—Jorge A. Gonzalez, M.D.
Co-Medical Director
HealthSouth Rehabilitation Hospital at Tulsa, Oklahoma

PREFACE

In one second, my whole life changed. One moment I was awake and alert; the next, I was involved in a head-on auto accident. Days later, my doctors diagnosed me as having suffered a mild head injury, now called mild traumatic brain injury (MTBI). At the time, this meant nothing to me, since I looked and felt fine save for minor cuts and bruises. All I wanted to know was when I could return to work.

In the months that followed, many of the signs of brain injury, or postconcussive syndrome, appeared. It took me years to understand the consequences of my mild traumatic brain injury. None of my doctors fully explained my problems, told me what to expect, or explained how to cope.

At first, I felt all alone. However, I soon discovered that there were local support groups for brain-injury survivors, as well as brain-injury associations in every state. Then I discovered the Internet, which opened a worldwide support system. Through on-line service providers such as Prodigy, CompuServe, America Online (AOL), and Microsoft Network (MSN), I have met hundreds of supportive people at all hours of the day. I discovered that each brain-injured person and situation is different and unique.

Having gone through the experience of MTBI, I know that while the causes of brain injury may differ, the ongoing consequences are the same. Survivors, family, and friends need help in the form of knowledge about postconcussive syndrome and how to cope with it. This book is designed to be a practical guide that allows you to focus on the specific things that affect you personally. Much of the information provided here may also be useful to people with acquired brain injury (ABI) due to stroke or brain tumors, since any type of injury to the brain can potentially cause similar consequences.

In addition to objective information, you will find information that comes from my own experience as well as that of other individuals who have survived MTBI. Although only their first names (or in my case, my initials) are used, all of the stories you will read are from real people. In addition, every chapter of this book has been reviewed by field experts to ensure that the information is accurate. The names of these experts appear in the Acknowledgments.

My recovery from MTBI has been slow. There have been many setbacks. Yet like many others, I am living proof that where there is a will, there is a way to move beyond the effects of brain injury. I'm not the person I was before my accident. Instead, I am a composite of the old and the new. However, I have learned that positive changes can take place if you understand the problems and know how to deal with them.

It is my hope that this book will answer your questions, help solve your problems, and give you hope for a productive life following mild traumatic brain injury.

–●–Diane Roberts Stoler
Georgetown, Massachusetts

A Word About the Mild Traumatic Brain Injury Label

Until recently, any traumatic damage to any part of the head or brain was called a "head injury." Since 1989, when the United States government earmarked the 1990s as the Decade of the Brain, extensive research has been done into all aspects of the brain, especially brain injury and its consequences.

In 1994, the World Health Organization adopted terms that are more descriptive of actual injuries to the brain. *Acquired brain injury* (ABI) is used to describe any damage to the brain that is not present at birth. A type of ABI, called *traumatic brain injury* or TBI, includes any damage to the brain that is caused by an external acting force. The ongoing long-term consequences of brain injury are called *postconcussive syndrome,* or PCS.

These changes led the National Head Injury Foundation to change its name to the Brain Injury Association effective July 25, 1995. On July 29, 1996, President Bill Clinton signed the Traumatic Brain Injury Act, which provides for expanded studies of and innovative programs for treatment of brain injury.

Throughout this book, we have chosen to use the current terms of mild traumatic brain injury (MTBI) and postconcussive syndrome (PCS) to describe what heretofore has been known as mild head injury.

About This Book

Within the next few seconds, someone in the world will incur a traumatic brain injury from an automobile accident, assault, fall, sports accident, or incident of physical abuse. Depending on his or her immediate symptoms, such as loss of consciousness, dizziness, or physical complaints, this person may or may not receive medical treatment. If he or she is unconscious for less than sixty minutes and appears fine afterward, the diagnosis will likely be mild traumatic brain injury (MTBI), and the individual will be told to rest at home for a few days or weeks.

This prescription of rest and time is indeed appropriate for many people with mild traumatic brain injury. However, many others encounter ongoing symptoms that continue to adversely affect their daily lives. These symptoms usually become apparent when people attempt to resume their responsibilities at home, work, or school.

This book is designed to help you understand and cope with the postconcussive symptoms that follow a traumatic brain injury. It is set up in five parts and contains a detailed glossary, as well as extensive reference and resource sections.

Part One contains information about the brain, the specifics of MTBI, and methods of diagnosis and treatment. Part Two details the various physical symptoms that can follow this type of injury. Problems with thinking are covered in Part Three, and the emotional repercussions of MTBI are explored in Part Four. Part Five addresses such related topics as financial, insurance, and family issues; rehabilitation; and eventual outcomes. In Part Two through Part Five, each individual chapter deals with one particular aftereffect of MTBI and provides a real-life story, an explanation of why the symptom or problem occurs, information on treatment, and practical suggestions for coping with the problem.

If you are reading this book, you probably already know that the effects of MTBI can be far-reaching as well as long-lasting. It is my hope that your recovery, or that of your loved one, will be made easier by the information, advice, and support included in the pages that follow.

PART ONE

MILD TRAUMATIC BRAIN INJURY— AN OVERVIEW

INTRODUCTION

Lynn, a 26-year-old dental hygienist, was driving to work one morning when her car was rear-ended at a red light. The fifteen-mile-per-hour impact caused no damage to either vehicle, and the seat belt kept Lynn's body in place. Only her head moved, quickly snapping forward and back. Lynn felt momentarily disoriented, but the feeling passed, and she went on her way without giving the matter much thought.

By lunchtime, Lynn had a severe headache. She discounted it as stress related. By evening, she also felt nauseated and extremely tired. At first, Lynn suspected a virus. But as the days passed, her headaches escalated and her fatigue increased. She also began to have problems sleeping, concentrating, expressing herself, and making decisions. To her patients, coworkers, and family, Lynn seemed uncharacteristically short-tempered and forgetful. Their continuing remarks to this effect led the puzzled young woman to see her physician. The eventual diagnosis? A mild traumatic brain injury (MTBI), a result of the months-ago incident at the traffic light.

Lynn's story is not at all unusual. In fact, each year more than 325,000 Americans suffer mild head trauma from falls, blows, collisions, sports injuries, and violent head movement such as whiplash. Like Lynn, a significant number suffer debilitating aftereffects for months or years afterward—despite a perfectly normal outward appearance. Part One of this book will help you better understand this phenomenon by providing a detailed look at the causes, significance, and evaluation of mild traumatic brain injury (MTBI).

1

WHAT IS
MILD TRAUMATIC
BRAIN INJURY?

In the course of everyday life, you have little reason to think about the workings of your brain. If you suffer a head injury, however, the subject takes on sudden importance. As with almost any injury, knowledge about the affected organ—the brain, in this case—will help you and your family to better understand your symptoms and maintain a sense of control over the recovery process.

A LOOK AT THE BRAIN

The human brain is the most complex of organs—an intricate network of some 200 billion nerve cells and a trillion supporting cells. The brain controls all bodily activity, from heart rate and movement to emotion and learning. It determines a person's abilities, personality, and state of health, and creates a capacity for thinking, feeling, imagining, and planning that exists in no other species.

While the human skull is hard and bony, the brain within has been likened to custard in a bowl—soft, pliable, and slippery. Directly beneath the skull are three thin membranes called *meninges* that hold pockets of air and about a coffee-cupful of *cerebrospinal fluid*, which cushion the brain. Directly beneath the meninges is the wrinkled, gray-white *cerebrum*, which caps the entire brain.

The cerebrum, sometimes called the *cerebral cortex*, is the largest and most advanced part of the brain. It controls problem-solving, planning, and judgment, as well as movement and sensory activity. It consists of veins, arteries, capillaries, and millions of threadlike nerve fibers. The cerebrum is divided into two halves, or *hemispheres*—the left and the right. One curious fact about brain function is that the

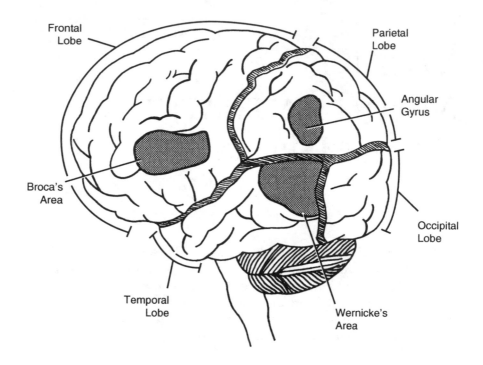

Figure 1.1 A Look at the Cerebrum

right hemisphere, or the right side of the brain, controls the left side of the body, while the left hemisphere controls the right side of the body. In addition, the right hemisphere governs aspects of creativity and nonverbal communication—gestures, facial expressions, and the like—while the left hemisphere is responsible for logical thinking and verbal and written expression.

Both of the hemispheres are subdivided into parts called *lobes,* each of which controls specific body functions. (See Figure 1.1.) The *frontal lobe,* located closest to the forehead, controls emotions and behaviors, social and motor skills, abstract thinking, reasoning, planning, judgment, and memory. *Broca's area,* situated at the base of the frontal lobe, helps to govern speech.

The *parietal lobe* is located halfway between the front and back of the skull. This area is responsible for sensory and spatial awareness, giving feedback from and understanding of eye, hand, and arm move-

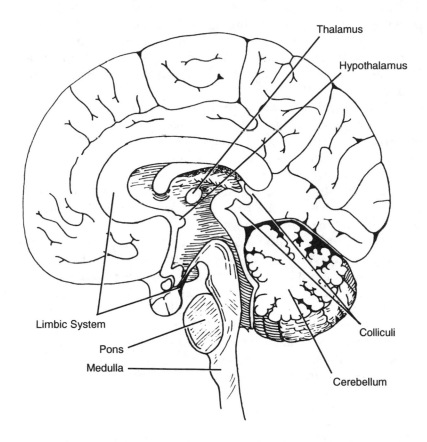

Figure 1.2 The Inner Structures of the Brain

ments during complex operations such as reading, writing, and numerical calculations. At the center of the parietal lobe is the *angular gyrus,* a fold in the surface of the brain where visual messages, such as words that are read, are matched with the sounds of spoken words. At the back of the head, behind the parietal lobe, is the *occipital lobe,* which controls vision and recognition.

The fourth brain segment, the *temporal lobe,* is located beneath the frontal and parietal lobes, and has an influence on emotions. The temporal lobe plays a part in smelling, tasting, remembering information, noticing things, comprehending music, and categorizing objects. It also plays a role in aggressiveness and sexual behavior. At the back of the left temporal lobe is *Wernicke's area,* which is responsible for hearing and interpreting language.

Beneath the cerebrum are a number of internal brain structures (see Figure 1.2). The *thalamus* acts as a nerve-impulse relay station for information coming into the brain, passing it to the *hypothalamus* to be prioritized and transmitted throughout the body. The hypothalamus also influences sex drive, sleep, long-term memory, and the expression of emotion. The *limbic system* helps the hypothalamus prioritize incoming information and also plays a part in controlling memory and emotion.

At the central rear of the brain is the *brain stem,* which contains the *midbrain,* the *pons,* and the *medulla oblongata.* These structures control breathing and heartbeat, and serve as a relay station for all motion and sensation. The *cerebellum,* a part of the brain situated in a cupped position slightly above the brain stem, oversees movement and balance, while the *hippocampus,* centrally located next to the temporal lobe near the base of the brain, is a key area in the transition of short-term to long-term memory.

Each part of the brain is highly specialized, and is able to do its job only because of its component nerve cells, or *neurons.* Each neuron consists of a cell body and a conducting fiber that can be as short as a fraction of an inch or as long as several feet. When working properly, these fibers transmit electrical impulses to adjacent nerve cells at speeds of up to several hundred miles an hour. In fact, a single healthy nerve cell can send impulses dozens of times per second. Damage a nerve-cell fiber, however, and you will disrupt the smooth flow of information to the receiving area within the brain.

TYPES OF INJURIES THAT CAUSE MTBI

Injury to the brain from an outside force, called a traumatic brain injury (TBI), can occur from a variety of causes. Automobile accidents, which account for approximately 50 percent of all cases of TBI, are the most prevalent cause. Other common causes of TBI include falls (21 percent); assaults and violence, including physical abuse (12 percent); and sports- and recreation-related accidents (10 percent).

There are two types of TBI: open-head injury and closed-head injury. In open-head injury, the skull is penetrated. Brain damage results in a focal injury—that is, injury to a specific area of the brain—such as that from a gunshot wound or external trauma that causes the brain to swell. In closed-head injury, the skull is not penetrated. Brain damage occurs as a result of an external force that causes the brain to move within the skull, producing both focal and diffuse, or generalized, injury.

The human skull and the underlying fluid-filled membranes rarely sustain damage during an MTBI. Any time the head is subjected to violent force or motion, however, the soft, floating brain is slammed against the skull's uneven interior. Sometimes it rotates in the process. When this happens, the brain's threadlike nerve cells are stretched and strained, and may even be torn, at the point of impact (focal injury) and/or in a widely scattered fashion (diffuse injury). Many times such an accident causes both stretching and tearing of nerve fibers. While this nerve-cell damage is usually microscopic, the effect on the brain's neurological circuits is quite significant.

Direct Contact Force MTBI

Impact injuries, or *direct contact force MTBIs,* result in observable tissue damage to a particular area of the brain. One common type of direct contact force injury occurs during car accidents and other incidents that involve acceleration followed by rapid deceleration (acceleration/deceleration injury)—that is, when the forward-moving head comes to a sudden stop after striking a stationary object. When this happens, the brain keeps moving within the skull until it makes sudden contact with the front of the inner skull. This causes *fronto-temporal lesions,* or bruising of the frontal and/or temporal lobes of the brain. (See Figure 1.3.) This type of injury generally affects a person's ability to memorize, plan, concentrate, and/or control behavior—skills that are largely regulated by the frontal and temporal lobes. You may have difficulty storing and retrieving new information, be unable to organize your thoughts, be highly distractible, or have problems modulating your behavior. These impairments result from disruption of the nerve connections between the cerebrum and the inner brain—in effect, a neurological short circuit.

A second type of direct contact force MTBI is the *coup/contrecoup* (literally, "blow/counterblow") injury. Generally, this trauma occurs when a moving object makes contact with the head, briefly denting the skull inward. The brain beneath is bruised first at the point of impact and then is thrown against the opposite side of the skull, where additional bruising takes place. (See Figure 1.4.) In coup/contrecoup cases, the sites of bruising and the resulting impairments depend on where the initial blow landed. You may encounter one or more of a range of problems, including personality changes, perceptual and sensory problems, difficulty expressing yourself, and balance and motor difficulties.

Diffuse MTBI

A mild blow to the head that causes momentary unconsciousness but no observable disruption of nerve impulses is called a *diffuse MTBI*

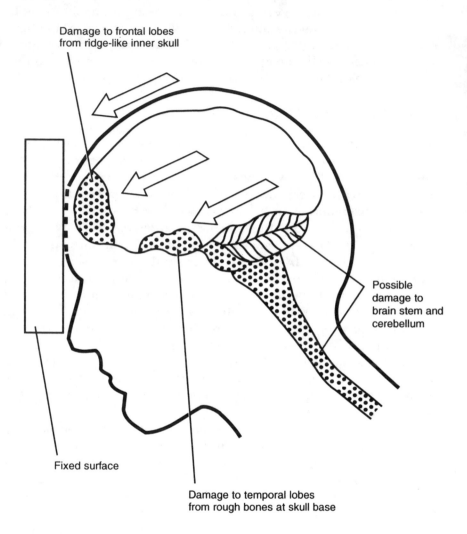

Figure 1.3 Acceleration/Deceleration Injury

In this type of injury, the head, which is moving forward, comes to a sudden stop when it hits a stationary object. When this happens, the brain keeps moving forward within the skull until it strikes the front of the inner skull, bruising the frontal and/or temporal lobes.

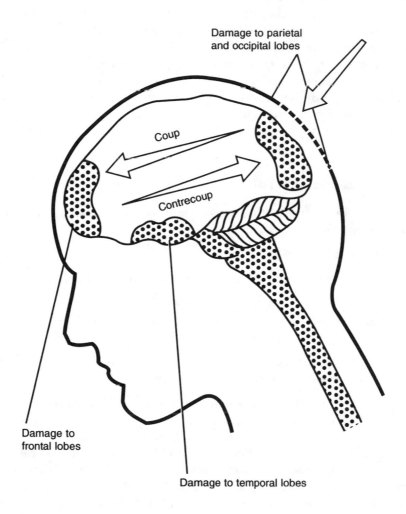

Figure 1.4 A Coup/Contrecoup Injury

In a coup/contrecoup injury, a moving object strikes the head, denting the skull inward and also knocking the brain against the opposite side of the skull. This results in bruising in two places within the brain: at the site of the original point of contact and the opposite side, where the brain struck the skull.

or *concussion.* (See Figure 1.5.) It was long believed that diffuse MTBIs caused only a brief short-circuiting within the brain. However, it is now known that the stretching of nerve cells due to movement of the brain in various directions at once interferes with their ability to fire impulses. This leads to loss of consciousness and, in turn, a general disruption of mental processes. People with diffuse MTBIs process information slowly, have trouble splitting their attention between tasks, and often find themselves struggling to organize and sort the details of incoming information. Abstract thinking may be impaired, as may the ability to express thoughts accurately and clearly. Diffuse MTBI can occur either alone or in conjunction with a direct contact force MTBI.

Secondary Causes of MTBI

Along with focal and diffuse nerve damage, MTBI can result from factors deemed secondary causes. These include:

• Anoxia, or a lack of oxygen.

• Contusion, a bruise that can go undetected during conventional testing.

• Edema, or swelling due to an accumulation of fluid in brain tissue.

• Hematoma, a localized brain swelling due to an accumulation of blood from a break in a blood vessel.

• Hemorrhage, or bleeding, in which a torn vessel releases blood into the brain tissue.

Most of the nerve cells affected by an MTBI sustain only relatively minor damage and eventually return to normal functioning. It is those cells that are seriously affected, or destroyed, by overstretching, tearing, bleeding, and/or swelling that ultimately shape an individual's postaccident experience. The brain is susceptible to even greater damage if repeated minor head trauma compounds an initial injury. Impairments like those sometimes exhibited by retired boxers and other athletes who have suffered successive concussions clearly illustrate this scenario.

DEFINING MILD TRAUMATIC BRAIN INJURY

Mild traumatic brain injury is characterized by a brief (or negligible) loss of consciousness and memory, with neither symptom lasting

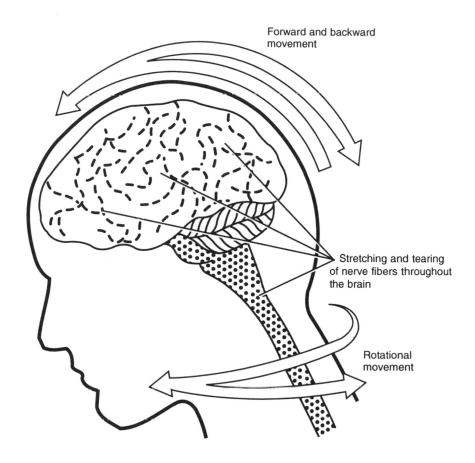

Figure 1.5 A Diffuse MTBI Caused by Whiplash

The rapid snapping back and forth of a whiplash injury causes the brain to move in two or more different directions at once, stretching and tearing nerve cells throughout the brain, rather than causing injury to any specific area.

Table 1.1 Common Consequences of MTBI

Type of Symptom	Examples
Physical	Fatigue
	Sleep disturbances
	Headaches
	Dizziness
	Nausea and vomiting
	Blurred vision
	Hearing problems
	Loss of sex drive
Cognitive (mental)	Distractibility
	Disorientation
	Temporary amnesia
	Short-term memory problems
	Poor judgment
	Slow thinking
Emotional	Depression
	Agitation
	Apathy
	Irritability
Behavioral	Confrontational attitude
	Explosive temper
	Fearfulness
	Impatience
	Thoughtlessness
Secondary psychological	Anxiety
	Fear of "going crazy"
	Frustration or anger
	Guilt or shame
	Feelings of helplessness

longer than sixty minutes. Many injuries of this nature cause only temporary disruption of brain function, and resulting problems fade within a week or two. This is due to spontaneous healing of brain and nerve tissue or the formation of new nerve-cell pathways that bypass damaged circuits. However, fully 60 percent of people who suffer an MTBI still encounter neurological problems three months after the injury.

Given the brain's susceptibility to injury from fender-benders, mis-fired fastballs, and other common hazards, you may wonder whether the term "mild" can ever really be used to describe a brain injury. The fact is that the word "mild" refers to the extent of brain trauma as indicated by responsiveness and recall. It does *not* describe the changes in thinking, behavior, and personality that many people find so difficult to cope with. A person who is briefly knocked out by a fall on the stairs is said to have suffered a mild traumatic brain injury even if she is plagued by a word-finding problem for years afterward. A child who suffers a concussion in a bicycle accident receives a similar diagnosis, even if he suddenly develops significant problems studying or paying attention in class.

The fact is that terms describing the severity of head injury are relative. A head injury is termed moderate or severe only if it involves penetration of the skull; prolonged coma; signs of deteriorating neurological status such as pupil dilation, breathing difficulties, and slowed heart rate; or evidence of localized brain damage such as speech or vision impairment. By practical definition, of the more than 2 million cases of TBI reported each year, only 22 percent receive hospital or other medical attention. Thousands of others go undiagnosed because no medical treatment is sought, despite troubling and/or persistent aftereffects.

CONSEQUENCES OF MTBI

Most people who have experienced severe brain trauma display language, motor, or perceptual problems that can be traced to a specific incident or event that caused a specific type of brain damage. The problems that result from MTBI are much more difficult to pin down. Some people suffer no ill effects at all. Others encounter persistent problems and feel the effects in every aspect of their lives.

In addition to suffering from head or neck pain, many people are disoriented and experience memory loss immediately after an MTBI. These complaints often pass within a few minutes, but over the next several hours the onset of dizziness, nausea, and fatigue is very common. A week or two later, as the individual attempts to resume his or her normal responsibilities at home, school, or work, he or she may encounter another group of symptoms that have collectively come to be called *postconcussive syndrome.* These complaints include persistent headaches; fatigue; impaired attention, concentration, and decision-making ability; sleep disturbances; dizziness; loss of sex drive; intolerance to alcohol; reading and communication difficulties; and emotional or behavioral problems. They may occur singly or in any combination. (A concise list of the most common MTBI symptoms and aftereffects can be found in Table 1.1.)

Whatever MTBI-related symptoms an individual experiences, they are likely to be compounded by social and psychological factors. For example, as the person with MTBI wrestles with a set of problems that affect every aspect of daily living, he or she often does so in secret. Because most MTBI problems are invisible to the casual observer, the injured person often hears such comments as, "You look just wonderful!" or "It's great that you're already back in the swing of things!" Of course, the person quite often isn't *feeling* wonderful at all, and is painfully aware of *not* functioning as he or she used to. This causes many people with MTBI to feel anxiety and lose their self-confidence, problems that can reveal themselves in out-of-character behaviors like self-involvement and extreme vulnerability to stress. Even worse is the fact that by the time the consequences of MTBI begin to disrupt an individual's life, he or she may not even relate the symptoms to the accident that caused them. It is no wonder, then, that after weeks of seeing little or no improvement in their symptoms, many people with MTBI find themselves faced with yet another roadblock—persistent depression.

Perhaps the greatest impact of MTBI is psychological. An unexpected, unexplained inability to function can deeply shake your sense of self. Consider the insurance agent who must suddenly struggle to remember clients' names and navigate the office complex; or the student who can no longer stay focused on classwork or note-taking; or the mechanic who can no longer reassemble an engine. None of these people looks any different than before. But they are all in trouble at work or school, and quite likely also are struggling to cope with everyday chores and concerns at home. Many people with MTBI begin to second-guess their every move in an attempt to avoid failure and embarrassment. This sort of anxiety can easily initiate a vicious cycle— it can build to such proportions that it actually contributes to the person's cognitive problems (problems with thinking, understanding, and reasoning), which in turn makes the anxiety worse, and so on and on.

Some people's MTBI-related symptoms fade away within a few weeks of injury. For others, the process takes longer. If the injury damages a sufficient number of brain cells, an individual may be left with permanent deficits. If a child suffers an MTBI, persistent aftereffects are often confused with developmental problems. Many thousands of people each year are misled by their "mild"—or missed—diagnoses.

If you are just beginning the process of recovery from MTBI, you should know that it is common to feel afraid and even, perhaps, as if you are losing your mind. After all, time has passed since your injury, you look just fine, and your diagnostic tests have all yielded normal results. Yet, clearly, all is *not* well. It will probably take a sympathetic doctor's referral and a neuropsychological workup—a diagnostic process designed to reveal problems with reasoning, memory, and other brain functions—to finally pinpoint the source or sources of your difficulties. Once that is accomplished, you will almost certainly feel an overwhelming sense of relief that someone understands what you have been going through. This affirmation, along with support from medical professionals, friends, and family, can help to head off many of the debilitating psychological responses to MTBI.

Overall, the outlook for recovery from MTBI is brightest with early diagnosis and treatment of symptoms. Optimally, you can hope for slow, steady progress toward normalcy in the months after injury. If it is determined that long-term or permanent cognitive deficits exist, you can best help yourself by understanding the nature of your problems, acknowledging your limitations, and making necessary accommodations at home, school, and work. The following two chapters will provide you with information about assessment techniques and the most successful approaches to lingering problems that can follow MTBI.

2

DIAGNOSING
MILD TRAUMATIC
BRAIN INJURY

Although most people who experience an MTBI appear quite normal within hours of the injury, new or lingering symptoms often compel them to seek medical assistance later. However, the definitive diagnosis that is needed to determine the best course of action can be elusive. Technology has only recently advanced to the point that the vague, diverse complaints that characterize MTBIs can be verified through diagnostic testing. In this chapter, we will look at the various methods and professionals involved in evaluating MTBI.

It is important to understand that conventional medical techniques are the only means of evaluating brain injury. No matter where your health-care preferences lie, any treatment of symptoms should always be preceded by a traditional diagnostic workup so that preexisting or potentially life-threatening conditions can be safely ruled out. Only with the most accurate possible diagnosis in hand can you make informed decisions about your postinjury health care.

THE CHALLENGE OF IDENTIFYING AN MTBI

"Your test results are negative. Go home, rest for a few days, and you'll be just fine."

For years, pronouncements like this were what people with MTBI typically heard after seeking medical help for symptoms such as dizziness, fatigue, headaches, memory loss, or distractibility. Doctors routinely disputed the existence of structural damage to the brain after MTBI because the diagnostic tools at their disposal were not sensitive enough to detect the nerve-cell damage that we now know can lead to a wide range of complaints. Traditional psychological testing also failed to pinpoint a problem, because the level of dysfunction of people with MTBI is subtle and their complaints are often nonspecific. So, since the possibility of an organic problem was dismissed and psychological tests were inconclusive, the majority of people with MTBI were told that their symptoms were psychosomatic. Worse, some people were accused of faking their problems for insurance or sick-leave purposes.

Unquestionably, MTBI has a psychological component. After all, the overall disruption of mental processes so common to this type of injury, combined with lingering physical complaints, can easily lead to out-of-character behavior and emotions. However, the pervasive sense of confusion and helplessness that people with MTBI experience strongly suggests that there must be a physical basis for their problems. As a result, the confirmation of actual brain damage is a primary concern. Besides helping to steer people toward appropriate treatment, confirming the existence of brain damage affirms that their experience is real and frees them from the accusation that they are just being lazy or making things up. Not surprisingly, then, the goal of proving that the brain has suffered physical damage is usually shared by the victim's family, and is becoming increasingly important to professionals who specialize in diagnosing and treating brain injury as well.

Yet neurological evidence of MTBI can be elusive, even with today's sophisticated diagnostic techniques. As discussed in Chapter 1, nerve-cell damage resulting from mild traumatic brain injury can be either widely scattered or confined to one or two areas of the brain. Whichever is the case, physical abnormalities in nerve-cell fibers are extremely difficult to detect because these structures are microscopically small and extremely complex, and because there simply are so many of them within the brain. The fact that nerve-cell damage can occur without more obvious signs of injury such as skull fracture, bleeding, or swelling serves to compound the diagnostic challenge.

Just as physical diagnostic tests can yield false-negative results, psychological evaluations may also be ineffective at assessing the lingering problems of a person with MTBI. Traditional psychological tests involve brief, structured tasks that are performed in controlled environments and that tap old learning skills one at a time. In contrast, the deficits experienced by people with MTBI usually occur under more normal circumstances—that is, in the face of everyday noise and visual stimuli—and have more to do with the ability to process and remember new material. For example, problems with planning and organizing are common complaints.

There is good news, however. Technological advances are making diagnostic tests more and more sophisticated, and increasing numbers of physicians are recommending neuropsychological evaluation—testing that measures different aspects of brain function under varying conditions. Both of these factors improve the odds of correct diagnosis.

THE ROAD TO DIAGNOSIS

Not all people who suffer head trauma or whiplash lose consciousness or receive medical attention immediately after the injury. However, MTBI professionals view an evaluation by an emergency-room physician as the best course of action after any blow to the head, because even momentary loss of consciousness can foreshadow impaired judgment and improper reporting of the incident. In addition, headaches, confusion, and blurred or double vision, also characteristic of MTBI, may place a person in jeopardy if he or she chooses to drive, perform delicate tasks, or return to the activity that resulted in the injury. Moreover, in a small number of cases, the individual's condition actually deteriorates in the hours after the accident because of brain swelling or bleeding. It is therefore wise to have any head injury evaluated as quickly as possible.

Parents and others who care for children need to know that if a child suffers a blow to the head, his or her condition immediately afterward is *not* a reliable indicator of how seriously the brain has been injured. Often, a coach or parent will brush off the fact that a child has been knocked out briefly during play. While in most such cases, children recover and are perfectly fine, it is possible for a child to have residual postconcussive effects from a seemingly minor blow to the head. If there is any doubt, or if a child exhibits behavior changes after injury, he or she should be seen promptly by a doctor with a background in MTBI.

The Initial Evaluation

In most situations, mild traumatic brain injury is an insult to the brain caused by external impact from a fall or blow, or by violent movement of the head. People with MTBI who receive medical treatment after injury are usually evaluated according to one or more of the following criteria to determine the existence and severity of brain injury:

- Any period of loss of consciousness during which there is no speech or meaningful response to touch and talking.

- Any loss of memory for events immediately before or after the injury.

• Any alteration in mental state at the time of the injury, such as feeling dazed, disoriented, or confused.

The label MTBI is given when unconsciousness or posttraumatic amnesia (memory loss following an injury) lasts less than an hour. An unconscious state that lasts longer than an hour is termed a coma. Memory loss that lasts longer than an hour is considered an indication of moderate to very severe brain injury, as follows: one to twenty-four hours, moderate; one to seven days, severe; longer than seven days, very severe.

An individual's overall responsiveness and potential for recovery are measured by the Glasgow Coma Scale, used primarily in emergency rooms and intensive care units. This scale measures awareness and assesses motor and verbal function and coma level (*see* The Glasgow Coma Scale, page 25). A score of 13 to 15 on the Glasgow scale is considered indicative of MTBI. A person who scores *lower* than 13 is considered to be moderately or severely injured. Interestingly, the Glasgow Coma Scale has been criticized by neurologists because it assesses a patient's condition at the time help arrives rather than immediately after injury. Many accident victims have already emerged from an unconscious or semiconscious state by the time police or medical personnel arrive. It is therefore easy to imagine that many brief blackouts—and the nerve-fiber damage that causes them—may be overlooked in the treatment of accident victims. As a result, a brain-injured person may be discharged from medical care with more severe neurologic problems than anyone realizes at the time.

About 12 percent of people who experience MTBI are hospitalized overnight for observation after injury. Most people, however, are sent directly home from the emergency room or doctor's office with nothing more than a prescription for rest and painkillers. Other times— as in the case of Lynn, the dental hygienist whose story was told in the introduction to this section—the injured parties themselves see no need for medical attention and dismiss their accidents completely until symptoms start to play havoc with their day-to-day functioning. A visit to a primary health-care provider or hospital emergency room may then lead to a skull x-ray, an electroencephalogram (EEG), or a computed tomography (CT) scan to check for skull fracture or brain injury. (More about these procedures later in this chapter.) Pain medication may be ordered for headaches. A person may also be referred to a neurologist (a medical doctor who specializes in disorders of the brain and nervous system) or other specialist for evaluation of persistent or additional symptoms.

The Glasgow Coma Scale

The Glasgow Coma Scale uses an individual's reactions to outside stimuli to assess the severity of brain injury. Medical personnel look for the level of response in three different categories, as detailed in the table below.

Best Response	Stimulus	Score
Opens eyes	Spontaneously	4
	In response to voice	3
	In response to pain	2
	Does not open eyes	1
Moves	In response to commands	6
	Examiner's hand away from pain site	5
	Body part away from pain site	4
	By flexing in response to pain	3
	By becoming rigid in response to pain	2
	Does not move	1
Verbalizes	In an oriented manner	5
	In a confused or disoriented manner	4
	Using inappropriate words or phrases	3
	Using incomprehensible sounds	2
	Does not verbalize	1

A person's total score equals the sum of the responses in each category, as assessed by a trained specialist. The score is then used to determine the severity of brain trauma as follows: 13 to 15, mild injury; 9 to 12, moderate injury; 3 to 8, severe injury.

Neurological Examination

A neurological examination is a workup done to assess a person's neurological functioning and look for signs of neurological injury. One type of neurological examination is performed on a large percentage of MTBI people by emergency medical technicians (EMTs) and emergency room doctors. Because most people who suffer MTBI are unconscious only momentarily (or not at all) and score well on the Glasgow Coma Scale (see above), they may receive only a cursory examination that measures alertness, attention, and general cognitive functions such as immediate recall. If there is a question of seizures or head trauma, then a specific diagnostic evaluation will probably be done immediately, and a neurologist may be consulted. However, if you can walk and talk, seem oriented, and answer questions correctly, you will likely be pronounced well based on your appearance and behavior. This is because many doctors lack firsthand experience with MTBIs and so prescribe only patience, rest, and pain medication. You may therefore miss the opportunity for an in-depth examination by a neurologist, despite troubling deficits that may soon interfere with daily living. Fortunately, some physicians are well enough versed in traumatic brain injury to pursue issues of thinking, reasoning, and memory dysfunction. Such a doctor will likely make a referral to a neurologist for an in-depth neurological examination.

An in-depth neurological evaluation has several parts. First, the neurologist obtains detailed information about the circumstances of the injury and resulting symptoms. He or she then takes a medical history, including family history, prior illnesses, injuries or infections, and information about such developmental milestones as walking, talking, and social skills. The neurologist also gathers information about hearing, vision, sleeping, work- or school-related interactions, and physical appearance.

Next comes a test of the cranial nerves. This provides information about vision, taste, facial expression, chewing, swallowing, balance, and the ability to speak. The neurologist may ask you to smile, follow his or her finger with your eyes, or listen for certain sounds during this part of the exam. Then he or she will assess components of motor function, including walking, the ability to stand on one foot, blinking, mouth movements, and eye-hand coordination.

If the neurologist suspects postconcussive syndrome, he or she will compile information regarding your alertness, attention, memory, reasoning, judgment, and understanding, and may request specific diagnostic tests to determine the nature of the suspected brain injury. In addition, he or she may refer you to a neuropsychologist (a psychologist with special training in the relationship between behavior and the brain) for an evaluation of your current level of functioning.

Neurodiagnostic Testing

This phase of the evaluation can include one or more x-ray, electrophysiological, and imaging tests. These are done to try to pinpoint the cause of postaccident symptoms. Your physician's decision for or against neurodiagnostic testing will probably depend on such factors as the length of time you spent unconscious and the severity of your head pain, disorientation, and memory deficits. Tests can be used to pinpoint damage to specific parts of the brain, thus giving both you and your doctor a better idea of what to expect in the way of a recovery process. The following are some of the neurodiagnostic measures most frequently used with MTBI patients.

Skull X-Ray

This two-dimensional picture of the head is usually taken from several angles to check for the presence of skull fracture after a head injury. This test photographs waves of low-level radiation as they pass through the affected area. The rays' passage is blocked by solid bone, which shows up as a white area on the developed film. However, x-rays easily pass through splits and cracks. If there is a fracture, it appears on film as one or more irregular dark lines.

The procedure is brief and painless—not unlike dental x-rays, except that the camera angle is different and you lie in a prone position to have it done. The disadvantage of a skull x-ray is that the test assesses only the brain's bony covering and yields no information about the functioning of the brain itself.

Electroencephalogram (EEG)

An EEG utilizes electrodes placed on the scalp to measure the electrical activity of the brain. Peel-and-stick electrodes are placed at strategic spots on the skull; at the other end, they are attached to a machine that displays and prints out results. A visual inspection of the EEG printout is done to assess the frequency and distribution of brain wave forms through various areas of the brain.

In MTBI cases, EEGs are used primarily to rule out such factors as seizure disorder or abnormal cell growth as the cause of neurological problems (or of the injury itself). The presence of abnormal brain wave patterns or slower than normal wave movement at any point during the test signals brain damage. Different versions of this test can be done on an outpatient, inpatient, overnight, or ambulatory basis. The test takes about twenty minutes and is completely painless. However, most people with MTBI have normal EEG results, so while the test may rule out certain conditions as the cause of your problems, it probably will not bring you any closer to a specific diagnosis.

Polysomnography

This test is an EEG recording that is performed while you are asleep to determine neurological changes, such as alterations in rapid eye movement (REM), frequent awakenings, or lack of dreaming. This test also provides information about restless leg syndrome, posttraumatic nocturnal seizures, and narcolepsy, conditions that can disrupt sleep/wake patterns, thereby causing fatigue and making other MTBI symptoms worse.

Quantitative Electroencephalogram (qEEG)

This diagnostic test is a computerized EEG that can detect not only breaks in and degeneration of nerve-cell fibers in the brain, but microscopic stretching damage as well. More sophisticated and informative than an ordinary EEG, the technique involves recording brain waves as signals played into a computer. The technician measures the time delay between nerve impulses moving about the brain as well as the time it takes for signals to be transmitted from one region to another. By comparing this information to certain standards, a specialist can often detect and diagnose a neurological basis for MTBI symptoms. The procedure takes about half an hour and is painless.

Computed Tomography (CT) Scan

This test, sometimes called a *computerized axial tomography (CAT) scan,* is based on x-ray technology. It is a three-dimensional imaging technique that shows much more detail than older techniques such as ultrasound and x-rays. A CT scan examines cross-sectional "slices" of the area in question and generates a series of screen images that can reveal masses, swelling, and/or bleeding within the brain.

The CT scan procedure takes about twenty minutes and uses a small amount of radiation. You lie on a half-cylinder, which moves slowly into camera range with a series of brief clicks. Dye is sometimes injected to provide a clearer image of the brain, and this occasionally leads to allergic reactions. (New, nonallergenic dye is available; however, the product is quite costly.) If you are highly allergic, your doctor may prefer to skip this test, since most people with MTBI do not sustain injuries severe enough to be detected by this technique. MRI, another three-dimensional imaging technique, outperforms the CT scan in detecting microscopic structural changes and other abnormalities of the brain.

Magnetic Resonance Imaging (MRI)

The MRI is one of the tests most frequently used to evaluate people with suspected MTBI. It uses computer technology and an intense electromagnetic field that acts on water protons in bodily tissue to project detailed images of the area under examination.

With an MRI, you lie horizontally in a metal cylinder for between forty and ninety minutes while the imaging is done. It is not unusual for the confinement, forced motionlessness, and external machine noise to cause anxiety, so you can usually opt to take a mild sedative before the test is begun. A so-called "open MRI" has recently been developed that all but eliminates the claustrophobia problem. Unfortunately, an MRI scan may be only marginally effective in detecting problems in nerve-cell tissue and body areas that contain little or no water.

Cerebral Angiography

This is a type of x-ray procedure that examines the structure of blood vessels and assesses blood flow to and within the brain. It is often done after a positive MRI to determine the type of structural damage present in the brain.

In this technique, you are placed in restraints to ensure that your head does not move. A thin catheter is inserted in a major artery and threaded through the arterial system to the beginning of the carotid arteries; then dye is injected. X-rays are taken as the dye makes its way to and through your brain. The procedure involves some discomfort, including soreness and bruising at the site of the catheter insertion and a burning sensation from the movement of the dye. As with all diagnostic tests involving dye, allergies can occasionally pose a problem. In addition, there is a small risk that a bit of plaque dislodged by the catheter may travel to the brain and cause a blockage or stroke.

Positron Emission Tomography (PET) Scan

This technique produces colored pictures of the brain's structure and function. It examines different areas of thinking activity, pinpoints the origin of seizures and other neurological problems, and evaluates any existing brain masses.

In this procedure, you are injected with a glucose (sugar) solution that contains a radioactive tag, which makes it possible to follow the speed and path of the solution as it travels throughout the brain. You lie prone on a thin table that moves slowly into a cylinder, not unlike the one used in a CT scan. Here, however, the machine is a receiver, feeding rays into a computer that analyzes data and eventually provides a three-dimensional image that is clear and precise—in effect, a picture of the brain at work. The PET scan detects irregularities in blood flow, nerve-cell activity, and the presence of oxygen. It takes approximately an hour.

The PET scan is a relatively new procedure and is used more for research than for clinical purposes. It is beyond consideration for many hospitals simply because they lack the funds to purchase the necessary machine—a quite-costly cyclotron. In addition, doctors may be reluctant to prescribe this test for patients who have had a number of CT scans because of the risks involved in repeated exposure to radiation.

Single Photon Emission Computed Tomography (SPECT) Scan

This procedure is similar to the PET scan in that it produces a three-dimensional image of the brain, although it is neither as expensive nor as precise. However, the SPECT scan does provide ready information about abnormalities and circulation within the brain. Its scan creates an image whose color and intensity reflect the amount of circulation activity present in that area of the brain, which can be compared to scans of other brain regions. Areas of damage show less or abnormal activity compared with that in the corresponding area of the opposite hemisphere. The SPECT scan can also be used to correlate the results of other procedures, including the MRI and neuropsychological tests. Together with the MRI and neuropsychological testing, the SPECT scan is one of the procedures most frequently used to evaluate people with suspected MTBI.

Other Diagnostic Procedures

In addition to the various tests described above, there are a number of other new, less often used tests that may be helpful in the diagnosis of MTBI. The *modal evoked potentials (MEP) test,* an electrophysiological study of the capabilities of the brain stem (see Chapter 1), is occasionally suggested, though it is more effective in screening more serious head injuries. The *transcranial doppler (TCD) test* diagnoses brain injury by viewing and assessing the flow of blood through six intracranial arteries. *Magnetoencephalography (MEG)* combines EEG and MRI techniques in assessing brain-wave movement and brain structure.

Neuropsychological Testing

In some cases, an exhaustive battery of neurodiagnostic tests fails to yield hard evidence of structural damage to the brain after MTBI. In other cases, repeat testing shows that signs of physical damage to the brain are improving, yet symptoms persist. At this point, it is often best to change directions—that is, to evaluate the extent, rather than the cause, of brain dysfunction. After all, you may have to live with your new limitations for some time. And regardless of the diagnosis (or lack of one), helping you cope with the injury's aftereffects should be the ultimate goal of all concerned.

A neuropsychological workup evaluates the effect of brain dysfunction on your emotional state, behavior, and mental functioning, and assesses discrepancies between your current and former skills and behavior. This evaluation provides a great deal of information about specific neurological deficits and the prognosis for recovery. The testing is done by a neuropsychologist who specializes in the emotional, behavioral, and cognitive problems that stem from brain dysfunction, and involves a careful review of your medical history and school and employment records. This is followed by a series of tests that measure a variety of cognitive and other skills, as well as various aspects of your personality and social behavior, under conditions that mimic those of normal living—that is, in the presence of constant new information and potentially distracting outside stimuli. A comprehensive neuropsychological examination takes between six and eight hours. Some of the tests that may be used include:

- *Intelligence tests.* These tests measure verbal and nonverbal abstract reasoning and general intellectual capability. Examples include the Wechsler Adult Intelligence Scale (WAIS) and the Wechsler Intelligence Scale for Children (WISC-R).

- *Academic skills tests.* These survey basic academic skills and reading comprehension. Examples include the Nelson Denny Reading Comprehension Test and the Wide Range Achievement Test.

- *Language skills tests.* These tests are designed to measure your ability to understand and use language. Examples include the Peabody Picture Vocabulary Test and the Boston Naming Test.

- *Nonverbal reasoning test.* This test measures the ability to establish, shift, and maintain thought processes. An example is the Wisconsin Card Sorting Test.

- *Visual perception skills tests.* These are done to evaluate the ability to perceive visual information. An example is the Hooper Visual Organization Test.

- *Memory tests.* These tests assess verbal and nonverbal memory skills. Examples include the Wechsler Memory Scale and the California Verbal Learning Test.

- *Personality tests.* These assess personality issues related to depression and anxiety. Examples include the Beck Depression Inventory and the Minnesota Multiphasic Personality Inventory.

The results of these tests are compared with your estimated level of functioning before injury and matched with your reported neurological symptoms. The relationships among the various deficits revealed during testing are also examined. This helps the psychologist to separate the effects of secondary problems, such as depression, from symptoms that are a direct result of brain trauma. Most important, this kind of evaluation can lead to specific suggestions about the treatment of symptoms—information that is much more useful than the general reassurances typically heard after a diagnostic workup. Neuropsychologists are perhaps the best source of information about rehabilitation and coping techniques, and can suggest approaches to recovery that are tailored to your particular needs.

DISSENT AMONG DIAGNOSTICIANS

Unfortunately, while today's technology and improved testing procedures have yielded welcome evidence that there *is* a physical cause behind MTBI symptoms, doctors and scientists still disagree on diagnostic procedure. One of the reasons for this is the small, but nevertheless significant, number of cases in which recovery from MTBI fails to correlate with test results and follow-up procedures. Sometimes, for instance, memory loss persists despite an improvement in the results of a patient's MRI. Or word-finding problems fail to fade at the same rate as signs of injury to the brain's speech centers. Circumstances like these lead to professional debate about many issues, among them the following:

- Are CT scans always a logical first step in the diagnosis of MTBI?

- Should MRIs and electrophysiological tests be used routinely?

- How far should diagnostic procedures be pursued when early exams are negative?

- How valid are the various tests as prognostic and follow-up tools?

- Do alternative practices like chiropractic, acupuncture, and natural remedies have a place in the evaluation of MTBI?

While some people may be unsettled by the experts' differing opinions about such issues, there are a number of valid reasons for their disagreements. For starters, different studies concerning the evaluation of head injuries yield different results. For example, a 1990 study measuring the validity of CT scans found that fully 18 percent of patients with Glasgow Coma Scale scores of 13 to 15—the range for MTBI— had abnormal test results. In fact, fully 40 percent of patients scoring

13 showed abnormalities. But a study conducted one year later found irregularities in only 3.5 percent of a similar patient group. In addition, studies sometimes overlook the importance of follow-up testing if initial test results are negative. This can cause doctors to be falsely confident about dismissing an MTBI patient's symptoms. Yet a 1991 study, for instance, found significant brain lesions twelve to twenty-four hours after injury in nearly 8 percent of patients whose earlier CT scans were negative.

The newer diagnostic techniques, such as brain imaging and electrophysiological tests, are time-consuming, costly, and available at only a relatively small number of hospitals. In today's tight financial climate, health-care professionals look carefully at the cost-effectiveness of such tests, which often involve not only the use of expensive equipment but also transporting the patient to a private facility some distance away. Particularly if you seem to be recovering at a more or less normal pace, your doctor may be unable to justify the expense of pursuing a specific diagnosis. He or she may also be hesitant about recommending alternative approaches, such as herbology and acupuncture, the effectiveness of which vary, and which have been subject to limited documentation and research.

Some medical professionals also question the effect on patients of doing every test available. There is a significant stress factor involved in many diagnostic procedures—they may be uncomfortable, and they raise the possibility of a discouraging diagnosis. For better or worse, therefore, physicians often guard against doing more testing than is absolutely necessary. Some practitioners may even hesitate to pursue testing that will spell out the precise causes of MTBI-related symptoms because of concerns that graphic descriptions of brain injury may lead to psychosomatic complaints that will hinder a patient's recovery.

Obviously, much more research is needed into brain function and the physical results of MTBI—and, hopefully, into finding a definitive procedure for evaluating MTBI. The improvement pattern among people with MTBI is not always consistent; memory deficits, problems with language, problem-solving difficulties, and other symptoms can be unpredictable. Ideally, people whose recuperation fails to follow the projected course will be able to gain hope from ongoing improvements in diagnostic techniques. With persistence, they may also find the missing pieces to their personal recovery puzzles.

3

APPROACHES TO
TREATING MTBI

Choosing an approach to treating MTBI—that is, finding ways to overcome and cope with the limitations imposed by such an injury—can be a great challenge. Whether or not a definitive diagnosis can be made, lingering symptoms can change your life for as long as they persist. You and your family will sense major differences in how you think and react, and it may soon become apparent that recovery will likely be a long, tedious process.

Fortunately, there are many different treatment approaches that may be helpful. In addition to a wide range of conventional medical therapies, such as drugs and physical therapy, there are also alternative treatment approaches that may be beneficial. Which treatment or treatments are right for you depends on the nature of your symptoms, your personal health-care preferences, and other factors. It is worth noting that no single treatment, whether conventional or alternative in nature, relieves every symptom for every person with MTBI. Nor does any particular combination of approaches guarantee a faster recovery from long-term problems with thinking, reasoning, and understanding. Circumstances and conditions are different for each case of MTBI. However, thorough evaluation, education, and the development of a strong support system are without exception the keys to progress in the months after injury.

To maximize your chances for successful recovery, you will want to ally yourself with a neurologist or other practitioner who specializes in treating brain injury, and who is nonintimidating, sympathetic, and, above all, willing to coordinate rehabilitation efforts with other health-care professionals. Once you have found such a professional, you and your family can turn your attention to choosing an approach or combination of approaches to wellness. As you do so, you should keep in mind that there are both physical and psychological sides to the aftereffects of MTBI. Slowly but surely, professionals in the field are arriving at the same conclusion: It is imperative to treat not only an individual's physical condition, but his or her cognitive (mental) function and emotional state as well. Treating the whole person appears to be the surest route to overall wellness.

CONVENTIONAL APPROACHES

The appropriate means of treating your MTBI symptoms depend on the kinds of difficulties you are experiencing and on your perspective on health care. There are several approaches to recovery that are commonly recommended by physicians. These techniques may be used individually or in conjunction with other treatments. Rehabilitative medicine and psychotherapy are two major approaches in this area.

Rehabilitation

This approach aims to return the person with MTBI to his or her former levels of functioning. Various types of practitioners provide rehabilitative services, including physical, occupational, and vocational therapists; speech/language pathologists; and special-education professionals. Rehabilitation can involve cognitive retraining—the relearning of skills in ways that make allowances for your limitations—or the approach can be educational, involving practice and exercises to gradually improve memory, visual and motor ability, concentration, and academic skills. Commonly recommended types of rehabilitative work include physical therapy, occupational therapy, vocational therapy, speech therapy, and special education.

Physical Therapy

This approach is often suggested for injury-related neck pain and whiplash injuries. A therapist trained in muscle rehabilitation guides you through a series of gentle exercises designed to decrease pain and strengthen the injured area. Massage and water therapy, in which water keeps the body buoyant and keeps pressure off the neck, are two popular techniques. Other treatments used by physical therapists include hot packs, ice massage, ultrasound, and therapeutic exercises.

Physical therapy and massage services are provided by licensed physical therapists, or LPTs, and by muscular or massage therapists, or MTs. An LPT has a bachelor's degree plus additional training in physical therapy and rehabilitative medicine. The LPT normally works under a physician's supervision in a private, school, or hospital setting, and is trained in anatomy, physiology, ultrasound, and muscular massage. In contrast, an MT works in a private setting and applies therapeutic movements to the muscles. Some training in anatomy is required for MT certification; training in rehabilitative medicine is not.

Occupational Therapy

This type of service is most commonly used with children, to help them build classroom and daily living skills. It can also be used to help brain-injured adults to improve their fine motor and social skills and to learn new techniques for managing everyday responsibilities such as shopping and household chores, as well as new ways of performing various job skills and how to avoid reinjury.

The registered occupational therapist (OTR-L) who provides this rehabilitation has an educational background similar to that of a physical therapist, but specializes in upper extremity rehabilitation. An OT aide or home health worker is able to assist the occupational therapist but is not specifically trained in rehabilitative techniques.

Vocational Therapy

This approach is most often used to evaluate past vocational or educational performance. Unlike occupational therapy, which increases a person's overall ability to function, vocational training targets a person's employment prospects, teaching new or different work skills and/or identifying job alternatives for those whose skills have undergone a change.

Vocational therapy is provided by a certified vocational counselor (CVC) or certified vocational educator (CVE). Such a practitioner has a bachelor's degree plus additional course work in employment retraining. A vocational therapist can practice in either a rehabilitation hospital or a private setting.

Speech/Language Therapy

This type of therapy helps to resolve communication and hearing disorders. A speech/language pathologist evaluates speech and language deficits and devises individualized therapy programs consisting of tasks and exercises to improve concentration, articulation, and listening and comprehension skills.

In order to be licensed and state-certified, a speech/language pathologist must have a master's degree with appropriate course work in the diagnosis and correction of speech problems. This professional can work in a private, school, or hospital setting.

Cognitive Remediation

This treatment is based on the premise that adapting to thinking, reasoning, and understanding deficits is less frustrating, and ultimately more successful, than reeducation. In cognitive remediation, you are helped to modify your environment to minimize the effects of your brain injury on everyday functioning. For instance, a job change, lighter course load, or reliance upon maps and lists might be recommended. You are also taught to remind others that you have difficulty recalling telephone numbers, screening out background noise, or whatever. This type of treatment is offered by rehabilitation psychologists with specialized training in health psychology and rehabilitative techniques.

Special Education

Special education is often used to help children find new approaches to academic work. However, adults who need to compensate for sudden neurological deficits can also benefit from evaluation and instruction in the use of computers and other "shortcuts." A special educator must have a bachelor's or master's degree in special education to be certified in most states. Special education is typically provided in schools and rehabilition hospitals.

Psychotherapy

Psychotherapy helps you to deal with behavioral or emotional problems and psychological reactions to life events. There are several types of, or approaches to, psychotherapeutic treatment. These include behavioral medicine, drug therapy, and traditional "talk therapy."

For psychotherapy following MTBI, it is important to select a mental health professional with knowledge of this type of injury. You may wish to consult a psychiatrist—a medical doctor who holds a state license and, in most cases, board certification in a specialty such as psychopharmacology (the use of medication to treat psychological disorders). A psychiatrist is licensed to prescribe medication and has expertise in the diagnosis, treatment, and prevention of emotional, behavioral, and mental disorders. Alternatively, psychotherapy may be performed by a psychologist, a state-licensed professional with a Ph.D., Psy.D., or Ed.D. degree, who may also hold board certification in a specialty such as behavioral medicine. A psychologist does not prescribe medication, but has training in cognitive and emotional assessment and the management of attitude and behavior problems.

Other types of practitioners who offer mental health services include clinical social workers, psychiatric nurses, and marriage and family counselors. A clinical social worker (LICSW) holds a state license and a master's degree, and may also possess board certification in a specialty such as geriatric care. A social worker does not prescribe medication but has training in family systems therapy and group therapy, as well as expertise in the diagnosis, treatment, and prevention of emotional and mental disorders.

A psychiatric nurse holds a master's degree in psychiatric mental health nursing and is certified as an adult clinical specialist (MSN RN CS). With special certification, a psychiatric nurse can prescribe and administer medication. The MSN RN CS has expertise in medical issues as well as the diagnosis, treatment, and prevention of emotional and mental disorders.

A marriage and family counselor, professional counselor, or marriage and family therapist needs no degree, though most have at least a bachelor's degree. The initials LMFCC, LPC, or LMFT following such a practitioner's name and degree refer to certification or licensing by state boards in that specialty. These counselors and therapists have expertise in family and marital issues.

Because it can be difficult to determine whether psychological symptoms are new or were present prior to injury—and because recommended treatments differ accordingly—psychotherapy for a person with MTBI should be provided only by a licensed mental health professional who has training in and experience with this type of injury.

Behavioral Medicine

This specialty treats specific aspects of medical complaints such as pain or muscle tension, and teaches better responses to these conditions. Behavioral medicine services should be provided by a board-certified psychologist (APPBM). One such technique, biofeedback, is performed by a specialist called a psychophysiologist. Biofeedback uses information gained by monitoring skin temperature, blood pressure, heart rate, and other body conditions to promote control over the normally involuntary nervous system through conditioning and relaxation. There are three types of biofeedback: thermal, muscular (EMG), and neurological (EEG). All employ some type of computer or monitoring device along with electronic sensors to give information about what is going on in the body. In thermal biofeedback, the device indicates physical changes like changes in pulse rate, body temperature, and breathing. EMG biofeedback indicates changes in muscular movement;

EEG biofeedback shows changes in brain-wave activity. These changes are displayed through visual graphs, sounds, or colors on a feedback display. Using these devices is something like looking in a mirror, but a mirror that shows your inner responses instead of your outer appearance. The appropriate type of biofeedback depends on the nature and causes of your symptoms.

Hypnosis, which is also very helpful for pain reduction, uses an altered state of consciousness to teach responses to and control over various trigger conditions. Psychologists who use hypnosis are board-certified in the use of the technique.

Traditional Psychotherapy

Traditional psychotherapy can help you to identify, understand, and cope with the symptoms and consequences of MTBI. There are various approaches to psychotherapy, each with its own theories and methods. Insight therapy, for instance, helps you to understand why things occur, while client-centered therapy provides you with an appreciation of yourself. Some therapies overlap. The use of role-playing and family counseling may be indicated as well.

The length, duration, and setting of psychotherapy depends on the individual's particular needs. As a rule, therapist/patient dialogue ("talk therapy") and stress-management training can be helpful to people with MTBI. Whatever type of psychotherapy you choose, it is important to select a mental health care provider who has special training in and experience with MTBI if possible.

Psychopharmacology

This facet of the psychotherapy field includes the use of medications to help change or regulate mental activity, mood, and behavior. Antidepressants and antianxiety agents are among the most commonly prescribed psychopharmacologic drugs. Among mental health professionals, only psychiatrists, who have medical degrees in addition to psychological training, can prescribe drug therapy. Psychopharmacologists are psychiatrists who specialize in the use of medications to lessen or eliminate psychological, neurological, and behavioral problems.

ALTERNATIVE APPROACHES

Conventional medicine is certainly the most familiar approach to health care, at least in this country. However, there are other approaches to wellness that are based on different perspectives on the interaction between mind and body. These alternatives, often referred to as "complementary medicine," do not necessarily oppose conventional medical wisdom. In fact, they are often used in conjunction with conventional approaches. For instance, acupuncture can be used to increase the effectiveness of pain medication. Alternative approaches are best tried after a diagnosis has been made through conventional means, and after conventional therapeutic approaches have been tried.

Most alternative approaches to coping with MTBI are individualized treatments that focus on natural healing of the whole person, not just correcting individual symptoms. As such, they can offer you additional paths to relief from lingering complaints, as well as a stronger measure of control over your recovery. The techniques discussed below have been used successfully by many thousands of individuals for such MTBI-related symptoms as head pain and cognitive difficulties.

Acupuncture

This practice uses the principles of traditional Chinese medicine, which focuses on the flow of the body's natural energy, or *qi* (pronounced "chee"), as a key influence on health. First, an evaluation is done, which may include questions and answers, pulse-taking, abdominal palpation, and examination of the tongue, skin color, and body odor. Based on the results of the evaluation, a treatment plan is devised involving the head and scalp, ears, or other part of the body. Hair-fine needles or topical herbal heat treatments may be used to stimulate points along the path of *qi,* thus helping the body heal through the harmonious flow of energy. One form of acupuncture, *auricular acupuncture,* involves gentle electrical stimulation of points in the ear.

The credentials of acupuncturists vary from state to state. Most states require at least a bachelor's degree, including premedical courses; some require two to three additional years of postgraduate work and a master's degree in acupuncture for a state license. The abbreviation L.Ac. or Lic.Ac. following an acupuncturist's degree indicates licensing, while Dipl.Ac. indicates board certification.

Chiropractic

This practice is based on the premise that pressure on nerves exiting the spinal column can cause neurological and circulatory problems throughout the body. Chiropractic involves manipulation of the spine to restore free movement and nerve functioning, thereby relieving a host of disorders and symptoms. This type of treatment is performed by licensed chiropractors, who are doctors of chiropractic and who have had four years of classroom and clinical training beyond college.

In cases of MTBI, a chiropractor may order an EEG, MRI, or other diagnostic test, in addition to cineradiography (a motion x-ray that determines the degree of trauma to the neck). This is done to rule out the possibility of problems that may result in further damage from certain treatments or movements. In addition to spinal manipulation, chiropractic techniques include soft tissue massage and stretching, as well as osseous (bone) treatments done with the hands or small tools. Techniques vary according to the type of injury, the practitioner's preferences and physical strength, and the patient's body type.

Homeopathy

This approach is based on the view that symptoms provide information about the body's attempts to heal itself. Homeopathic treatment involves the use of remedies made from naturally occurring substances that would create particular symptoms if taken in large amounts, but that stimulate healing of those same symptoms if taken in minute amounts in a highly diluted form. Before prescribing treatment, a homeopath evaluates symptoms according to their placement on certain mental, emotional, and physical planes. He or she will listen and observe as you speak in general about the influences in your life, and will be interested in minute details of your symptoms. How you present this information is as significant to the practitioner as what you say. Upon evaluating your symptoms, a homeopath will prescribe a remedy or combination of remedies to stimulate your body's natural self-healing capacity.

Only three states—Arizona, Connecticut, and Nevada—have specific licensing boards for homeopathic physicians (D.Hts.). Other states require homeopathic practitioners to have some form of certification or course work, though guidelines and requirements vary widely. It is wise, therefore, to inquire about credentials before working with a homeopath.

Herbology

Herbology combines age-old insight into healing with modern pharmacological research. An herbalist will assess your symptoms and treat them with herbal remedies that are tailored to your individual needs—prescribing relaxing herbs for muscle tension or severe headaches, for instance.

Herbal medicines originate from plants and often involve boiling the selected leaves, roots, and/or bark into soup or tea form. Today, many herbs are also prepared in tincture (a concentrated extract), powder, or pill form. No specific academic training is required of herbalists, though some states offer optional certification programs. We recommend that you thoroughly check the experience of an herbalist before taking his or her advice.

Polarity Therapy

This type of therapy is based on the Eastern philosophy that everyone has an "internal blueprint" that controls everything from personal achievement to healing. The goal is to identify blockages of internal energy and treat the resulting symptoms by placing you in better touch with your internal blueprint. Once back in balance, the body can better heal itself.

A typical polarity therapy session lasts forty-five minutes to an hour, during which you lie on a polarity or massage-type table and a therapist uses therapeutic touch to increase your relaxation response and hasten healing. Polarity therapists should be certified by the American Polarity Therapy Association (see the Resources section beginning on page 281).

CHOOSING A TREATMENT APPROACH

When considering your health-care options, you should thoroughly research any and all treatments or approaches, whether conventional or alternative. You need as much information as possible about procedures, costs, risk factors, and projected results in order to make informed choices. It is wise to consult with other people who have MTBIs about their opinions and experiences. While no two people should expect the same recovery experience, it is a good idea to find out what is (and what is not) working for friends and support-group contacts. Ask prospective practitioners about the possibility of contacting other patients or clients under their care to learn about their experiences. Additional information about people's experiences can be found through a local brain-injury support group as well as on-line bulletin boards, newsgroups, chat areas, or websites.

Finally, be prepared to be flexible. If you give an approach a fair trial without experiencing any improvement, or if you feel that a practitioner is either unsympathetic or underinformed about MTBI issues, you are justified in looking elsewhere for help.

FINDING THE RIGHT PRACTITIONER

Securing the services of the best practitioner or practitioners to treat your MTBI-related symptoms can be quite difficult because of the number of options available and because initial evaluations and treatment are often done in a crisis situation over which you have no control. However, the selection of the right professional can have a significant impact on the length and speed of recovery from lingering symptoms.

Once you have received a tentative diagnosis of MTBI and you have decided upon an appropriate path toward recovery, the next step is to find someone in the chosen area who specializes in treating people with MTBI and their unique symptoms. Doing so will guarantee a more refined diagnosis and, in many cases, more immediate relief from lingering discomfort or problems. The guidelines that follow can facilitate the decision-making process:

• Ask your primary health-care provider (the family physician or other practitioner who sees to your routine health-care needs) for advice and referrals. He or she can make recommendations based upon research into the treatment of head injuries, your medical history, and, possibly, familiarity with the practitioner or practitioners you are considering. This advice can be invaluable.

• Make a point of seeking practitioners who have a thorough understanding of, and experience with, MTBI and its symptoms. Always interview a prospective doctor or other practitioner to find out about his or her attitude toward and experience with the treatment of MTBI symptoms. (*See* Assessing a Practitioner's Expertise With MTBI, page 45, for a list of suggested questions to ask.) When dealing with MTBI, your health-care providers' expertise can directly affect the outcome of treatment.

• Look for practitioners who are open to cooperating and coordinating treatments with professionals in other areas. This is particularly important if you are interested in pursuing alternative treatment approaches. Physicians are often skeptical about such things as herbology or acupuncture, or even chiropractic treatment or the use of nutritional supplements. Yet many of the most successful recoveries are the result of a team approach, in which a number of professionals cooperate out of concern for all aspects of the patient's health.

• Include key family members in the process of choosing a practitioner or practitioners. Be aware that brain trauma can interfere with your judgment and reasoning. It helps to have someone else who can be objective assist you with decision-making.

• Consider taking advantage of a referral service that can provide helpful details and direct you to many conventional and alternative treatments. (See the Resources section beginning on page 281.)

Assessing a Practitioner's Expertise With MTBI

Research into the lingering aftereffects of MTBI is a relatively new field. As a result, many doctors and other specialists lack expertise in diagnosing and treating the varied and sometimes elusive symptoms of this sort of injury. However, you are more likely to experience a complete recovery under the treatment of someone who has training and experience with MTBI.

The following are some suggested questions to help you determine a prospective practitioner's level of expertise with MTBI:

- How many cases of MTBI have you personally been involved with in the past three years? *If the practitioner lacks experience with MTBI, look further.*

- What percentage of your practice is devoted to MTBI patients? *Thirty percent or more is optimal. Less than 5 percent means that you should continue your search.*

- Have you attended any seminars or conferences during the past two years that involved MTBI? *Ideally, the answer should be yes. If it isn't, do not continue with the practitioner.*

- Have you written any articles on MTBI in the past three years? *If the answer is yes, ask what type of article. Publication does not necessary signal good clinical experience.*

- Which textbooks do you refer to for information about MTBI? *Check the publication dates. Developments in the field are ongoing. Your practitioner should have the most current volumes.*

- Do you subscribe to "TBI Challenge" magazine, "Head Injury Update," "Headlines" magazine, "The Perspectives Network" magazine, and/or any other periodicals about brain injury? *Subscription to a TBI journal or magazine does not necessarily reflect a practitioner's competence, but it is desirable.*

The greater a practitioner's interest in and recent experience with MTBI, the better prepared he or she will be to assess your symptoms and prescribe and monitor your treatment.

As further study is done into the nature, range, and duration of MTBI aftereffects, the medical community is becoming increasingly aware of the broad scope of this type of injury. Each MTBI is unique. This makes both a tailor-made recovery approach and a diligent search for the right professional team imperative. In the chapters that follow, we will look in detail at many of the specific symptoms that are often seen in individuals with MTBI, along with the types of treatment approaches that have been shown to be helpful for each one.

PART TWO

PHYSICAL ASPECTS

INTRODUCTION

Terrie had been working for four months as a residential specialist at a transitional home for adults with traumatic brain injuries in Maine. She performed the duties of teacher, counselor, driver, accountant, friend, and referee, and learned a great deal about brain injuries. But then an auto accident taught her a great deal more.

On a rainy August morning, a squirrel ran in front of her car, which was traveling at about thirty miles per hour. Terrie jammed on the brakes, and her car hydroplaned and spun around three times before coming to rest against a rock wall. While the car was spinning, Terrie's body twisted and her ear struck the side window, but she was able to get out of the car afterward to assess the damage. When she did, onlookers and a police officer noticed that she was swaying, and she complained of dizziness and neck pain.

Terrie doesn't recall the ride to the hospital. She was told later that she lost consciousness. After undergoing x-rays and some observation, she was sent home—even though she could barely walk. In the weeks that followed, Terrie slept a lot and was in pain most of the time. She experienced headaches, hip pain, blurred vision, dizziness, fatigue, and numbness from her neck down into her arm. Her head felt as if someone were poking an ice pick into her left ear. The doctor she consulted never mentioned a brain injury, instead commenting that she looked fine. After Terrie spent two weeks on pain medication, the doctor extended the prescription for another month and a half, and recommended that Terrie go on disability.

The pain medication caused Terrie to become further disoriented and hysterical. The doctor agreed that the medication should be discontinued and prescribed physical therapy for her neck. He ignored her head, ear, and hip discomfort, though the physical therapist later pressed him to write orders for additional treatment. Terrie eventually underwent painful traction treatment.

Six weeks after her accident, Terrie met a doctor of osteopathic medicine (DO), who told her that her problems stemmed from postconcussive syndrome. Ironically, despite this very telling diagnosis, Terrie was eventually fired from her job because she could no longer drive. She comments that people with MTBI are the true walking wounded—they look just as they did before, but have changed a great deal.

Because the symptoms of MTBI, called postconcussive syndrome (PCS) seem in such contradiction to an individual's outward appearance of well-being and good health, there is a need to understand and learn how to cope with the many limitations that can be imposed by this type of injury. Happily, there are several avenues through which this can be accomplished—among them education, conventional medical treatment, alternative approaches, and lifestyle modifications.

Part Two of this book covers specific physical symptoms and consequences of MTBI. We present information about the nature of each problem, why it occurs, and how it can be identified and treated. This will help you and your family to understand what you are experiencing, and to make informed choices about treatment.

4

FATIGUE

Gail, a 45-year-old marine biologist from Oregon, was broadsided while driving home from work one day, and she struck her head. Weeks after her accident, she found herself struggling to live hour to hour, rather than day to day as in the past. Even going to the bathroom seemed like an ordeal.

Gail points to fatigue as the biggest problem she faces as a result of her MTBI. Because she is tired all the time, her possibilities for rehabilitation are severely limited. Gail has noticed that when she is tired, she doesn't cope well, sleep well, see well, or even speak properly. Her speech is slurred, and she frequently trips up the stairs.

Gail's fatigue is worst during fine motor activities. In fact, writing a single check exhausts her more than scrubbing floors. She explains that while floor-scrubbing requires her to fill a bucket and make large arm motions, check-writing calls for writing on lines, forming letters and numbers, knowing the date, and folding and inserting checks in stamped, addressed envelopes. Gail says that writing a check causes her to break out in a sweat, as if she were running a marathon.

Gail wonders how to explain to other people that she has a disability that does not affect her outward appearance, but that does keep her from doing things she once was able to do. It is very difficult for her to convince others— and, at times, herself—that her debilitating fatigue is a real consequence of her MTBI.

When you have had an active day or a later-than-usual night, the sleepy, yawning feeling that follows is a signal that your body needs rest. The fatigue that so often accompanies MTBI is very different. MTBI fatigue fogs your mind, saps your energy, deadens your limbs, and brings on an overwhelming need to sleep whenever and wherever the feeling strikes. The sleep you crave is often elusive and fragmented, however, and does little or nothing to relieve your bone-weariness and state of confusion.

Fatigue occurs three times as often among brain-injured people as it does among the uninjured population. Yet it is initially less noticeable than, say, balance problems or chronic headaches. As a result, it is frequently overlooked as an injury aftereffect. It is also easily misidentified. MTBI fatigue is particularly easy to overlook during the initial recovery period, when you are likely to rest frequently as you nurse your visible injuries. However, once you attempt to resume your previous pace, your sleep-defying exhaustion quickly becomes apparent.

WHY FATIGUE CAN OCCUR AFTER MTBI

Much research has been done on both acute and chronic fatigue, but it remains unclear why people often have no reserve energy or "second wind" after a brain injury. It is not known whether there is simply no energy left to use or whether the brain is unable to access it. However, we do know that once a person with MTBI uses up his or her energy, it takes longer to recharge than in the past—up to several days, in many cases.

You may feel extraordinarily tired if your MTBI affects your ability to fall asleep or disrupts your customary sleep/wake cycle. This is a common complaint, because sleep patterns are fragile and can easily be affected by brain injury. Particularly in the first four to six weeks after injury, pain and other symptoms may play havoc with two key facets of sleep: *sleep initiation* (your ability to fall asleep) and *sleep maintenance* (your ability to stay asleep). Often, people with MTBI awaken several times each night for no apparent reason.

Sleep problems may stem from *instrinsic sleep disturbances,* problems such as sleep apnea or narcolepsy that were present before the injury but that may be worsened by brain trauma. Or you may experience *extrinsic sleep disturbances,* which are environmental disruptions of sleep patterns due to things like pain, noise, or temperature that you would have been able to ignore in the past. Circadian-rhythm disturbance, or interference with the inner clock that regulates periods of sleep and wakefulness, may also be a factor. Circadian-rhythm problems may predate an MTBI but be worsened by it, or they may be caused by the injury. Common manifestations of this type of problem include night terrors, nightmares, or the kicking and twitching of restless leg syndrome.

WHAT MTBI-RELATED FATIGUE IS LIKE

"Prior to my MTBI, I maintained a very busy day. I would rise at 7:00 A.M.,

get my children off to school, go to the gym for two hours, have lunch, see five or six patients a day, and do supervision. After dinner, I would spend time with my family and end the night by writing progress notes on my patients until 11:00 P.M. Even at that hour, I had enough energy left to play my guitar and talk on the phone with friends.

After my MTBI, I spent the first two months sleeping nineteen hours a day. When I was up, I felt very fatigued all the time. Currently, my energy is limited to the hours between 8:00 A.M. and noon. By 1:00 P.M., the fog starts rolling in, making me feel inefficient or, at worst, spacy. By 3:00 P.M., my day is virtually over."

—D.R.S.

The fatigue that follows MTBI is lethargy in its most extreme form. It affects all aspects of your thinking, your physical abilities, and your emotional ability to cope with life. Many people with this type of fatigue first suspect a virus or a bad case of burnout, particularly if they fail to connect their exhaustion with other MTBI symptoms like headaches or neck pain. You may feel completely drained, as if you cannot make it through the day. Because fatigue affects your brain's ability to integrate information, your thoughts and responses may be as sluggish as your movements. You sense that you have lost your mental stamina—that is, your power of concentration, your memory, and your sense of motivation. Your moods may also be affected, because frustrations mount—and your ability to deal with them diminishes—as your efficiency and productiveness decline. Your ability to coordinate movements like walking and driving may be severely affected as well.

Like many people who have suffered MTBIs, you may find yourself battling your exhaustion with frequent naps, caffeine, and lots of carbohydrates and sugary snacks. But these and other tactics, which provide an energy boost under normal circumstances, now fail to bring on that second wind. The energy reserves that you normally depend on have suddenly vanished. Instead, you are likely to find that it takes several days to recover expended energy and that you have just a few "good" hours a day—usually in the morning. If you try to push your body beyond its new limitations, you may well experience something akin to circuit overload: An uncontrollable heaviness comes over you, as if you were being piled with lead weights; the need to lie down and rest is overwhelming; mental exhaustion leaves you confused, spacy, and faint; and the smallest frustrations make you feel emotionally wrung out. This opens the door to other emotional responses, such as grief over your lost or diminished abilities (this will be covered in detail in Chapter 21). Additional symptoms may follow, including insomnia, headaches, sexual dysfunction, depression, and/or irritability.

DIAGNOSING FATIGUE

It is easy to confuse MTBI-related fatigue with other conditions, including chronic fatigue syndrome, posttraumatic stress disorder, and various sleep disorders. Pervasive fatigue also shares symptoms with clinical depression, among them loss of appetite, insomnia, and chronic drowsiness. However, research has found no correlation between clinical depression and MTBI-related fatigue, except in people who have had previous problems with depression.

Sometimes, the fatigue that follows an MTBI is chronic, or ongoing. In other cases, it can strike in an acute form at unpredictable intervals. When you seek medical help, your doctor is likely to start by taking a thorough medical history. Because fatigue can be a symptom of so many different physical problems, the conclusion that your exhaustion is due to MTBI may be reached only through a process of elimination.

TREATING MTBI-RELATED FATIGUE

The time-honored approach to treating fatigue is to isolate and eliminate the cause rather than focusing on the symptom. Of course, this can be extremely difficult to do when MTBI is the culprit, since the exact nature of these injuries is so hard to pin down. Choosing an approach to treating MTBI-related fatigue is further complicated by the fact that treatments for many other MTBI-related symptoms can induce tiredness on their own. Many medications, for instance, have the side effect of causing fatigue, and the physical toll taken by various therapies can easily compound your existing exhaustion. However, many people with MTBI have overcome, or at least reduced, bothersome levels of fatigue by trying one or more of the conventional and alternative approaches described below.

Conventional Approaches

Many doctors try to reduce or eliminate fatigue with medication. There is no prescription medication available for general fatigue; however, substances designed to treat other conditions can sometimes bring a measure of relief, particularly if insomnia or depression is involved. In prescribing medication to combat your exhaustion, three factors must be taken into account: your postinjury tolerance for medication, the duration of the effects of different drugs, and the timing of dosages. After all, you wish to duplicate a normal daily cycle of alertness and drowsiness. A drug that keeps you either wide-eyed or mildly sedated around the clock is not very helpful.

Sometimes, sleep problems are treated with benzodiazepines, a class of antianxiety drugs divided into long-acting, intermediate-acting, and ultra-short-acting groups, depending on the duration of their effects and the speed of their absorption into the body. Some well-known examples of this type of drug include chlordiazepoxide (Librium), diazepam (Valium), alprazolam (Xanax), and triazolam (Halcion). Low-dose antidepressants may also be used for sleeping problems, although these medications may have side effects that can end up worsening such symptoms as daytime fatigue and memory difficulties. Commonly prescribed medications in this category include trazadone (Desyrel), doxepin (Adapin, Sinequan), and amitriptyline (Elavil, Endep). It is important to note that people with MTBI may be unusually susceptible to the sedating side effects of many types of medications prescribed for other health problems, including anxiety, depression, pain, and high blood pressure.

Dietary modifications are another approach to treating fatigue. Your doctor is likely to recommend that you avoid alcohol, caffeine, artificial sweeteners, and tobacco products, since these substances can play havoc with your stamina. High-energy foods that have undergone a minimum of processing are likely to be helpful. These include fruits, vegetables, whole-grain breads and cereals, dried beans, fish, and chicken. Your doctor may also recommend low-level regular exercise to be done at the time of day when you have the most vitality.

Recent studies have shown that EEG biofeedback and neuro-biofeedback can be effective for fatigue related to MTBI. A psychophysiologist, a psychologist trained in biofeedback techniques, can administer this kind of treatment. If you are unable to find a psychophysiologist in your locality, you can obtain a referral from the Association for Applied Psychophysiology and Biofeedback (see the Resources section beginning on page 281).

Alternative Approaches

Acupuncture, done by a licensed acupuncturist, can be helpful in combatting fatigue. Long-term relief from chronic exhaustion has been reported after as few as six acupunture treatments.

There are a variety of homeopathic remedies and herbal preparations that are advertised as energy boosters, among them the herbs ginkgo biloba and gotu kola. However, these over-the-counter products are designed for the general population, not as remedies for specific physical conditions and disorders. Moreover, each MTBI is unique. We therefore recommend that you consult with an appropriate and skilled practitioner before you use any over-the-counter herbal or homeopathic products. He or she can then recommend an alternative remedy or remedies especially suited to your individual symptoms and needs. If your physician is unable to help you with this or to provide an appropriate referral, organizations such as the Herb Research Foundation and/or the National Center for Homeopathy (see the Resources section beginning on page 281) may be able to help.

There are also nutritional and dietary supplements, such as bee pollen and vitamin B_6, that are claimed by some to increase energy and combat fatigue. Unfortunately, nutritional supplements and such products as melatonin, used to induce sound sleep, generally appear to have no significant effect on the type of ongoing fatigue that is characteristic of MTBI.

PRACTICAL SUGGESTIONS

"I've learned to cope with my fatigue by doing my writing or other thinking activities in the morning, when I have more energy. On my worst days, I cook dinner at noontime for my family or have my sons Brad and Alan do the cooking. One afternoon a week, I update a grocery list that I store in my computer, and shop with my youngest son, Alan. He helps keep me on track at a low-energy time of day."

—*D.R.S.*

As we have seen, MTBI fatigue has several different aspects. Each of them deserves attention during the treatment process. Sleep disruption may be the underlying cause of your exhaustion. Lost energy reserves may be the problem. Perhaps it is mental fatigue that troubles you the most. Or you may find yourself struggling with two or three of these problems. The following are a number of tried-and-true tactics to help combat each facet of fatigue. You may wish to experiment with a few of these suggestions to see which ones best help you maintain control over this bothersome symptom:

- To fight sleeping problems, go to bed at a set time every night, regardless of how you are feeling. Allot at least six but not more than ten hours for sleeping each night, and make it a point to rise at the same time every day, whether you have slept well or not.

- Limit your intake of fluids after 8:00 P.M. to avoid having your sleep disturbed by a full bladder.

- Avoid taking naps if possible. Brief snatches of sleep can play havoc with your body's ability to get a full night's rest.

- If your fatigue is overwhelming, try taking one midday nap to take the edge off your exhaustion. If your fatigue is extreme, this may help you sleep better at night.

- Take pain medication as prescribed to minimize the possibility of interrupted sleep.

- To cope with physical fatigue, organize your daily activities according to a priority list. This way, by the time you become fatigued, your most important responsibilities will have been taken care of.

- Avoid getting overtired. This can set you back for days. Pace yourself, take frequent rest breaks, and solicit the help of others.

- Vary your activities to avoid monotony, but do not try to tackle more than one task or activity at a time.

- To combat intellectual and emotional fatigue, avoid excessive stimuli such as sound and light. For instance, do your shopping by phone from home instead of subjecting yourself to crowded department stores. If you must go out shopping, do so when stores and roads are relatively quiet—say, at 10:00 A.M. or 2:00 P.M.

- Enlist your family's help in making your home a quiet place. Take a break from entertaining, turn down the telephone, and keep background noise to a minimum. Limit visitors to one or two at a time, and keep visits brief.

- Acknowledge your limited thinking capacity, and use it wisely. Schedule activities that require concentration for times when you are freshest. Research has shown that our thought processes tend to be clearer between 8:00 A.M. and 12:00 noon, and again between 6:00 and 8:00 P.M. Conversely, the hours of least efficient mental function are in the area of 3:00 A.M. and between 1:00 and 3:00 P.M.

- Ration your mental energy carefully during a week that contains a big event.

- Use shortcuts. For instance, prepare a general grocery checklist on which you need only add or delete items. Ask a family member to draw simple maps of the places you need to go. Combat memory problems with a pocket-sized tape recorder, math problems with a calculator.

- Take periodic rest breaks. If you feel a wave of fatigue coming on, sit or lie down and relax.

MTBI fatigue strikes different people in different ways. That physically leaden feeling, that frustrating loss of focus, and the inability to get a decent night's sleep are all common aftereffects of brain trauma. These problems can occur individually or in any combination.

Recovery from MTBI fatigue, which typically takes six months to a year, usually begins with a slow, sporadic return of surplus energy. As with many symptoms, you will start to have good days—but you will have occasional relapses that are difficult to predict. Often, the reappearance of a mental second wind in the early evening will be the first sign that your fatigue is beginning to abate.

There is no simple cure for fatigue, but using appropriate medication, modifying your surroundings and activities, and rationing your stores of energy can bring relief and a welcome sense that you are regaining control of your life.

5

HEADACHES

Barbara was a passenger in a car that was struck head-on by another vehicle. She was thrown forward into the windshield, then backward, and eventually out the car door. She spent weeks in the hospital because of her bodily injuries, but was also diagnosed as having an MTBI.

Barbara suffered recurring mild headaches for many months after her accident. Ten years later, she began to experience agonizing head pain after exertion or an increase in her body temperature. Any activity that caused her to perspire also produced a massive throbbing in her head, along with projectile vomiting. The pain continued long after she cooled down from her exercise. Naturally, Barbara has long since given up most sports and aerobic activities.

Sometimes, though, overheating can't be helped. Through trial and error, Barbara has found that taking some apple juice or Gatorade and lying down with an ice pack on her head interrupts the pattern and nips headaches in the bud. She has also found that activities that keep her head and body at an even temperature—swimming, walking on cool days, and skiing without a hat, for instance—enable her to exercise without pain. Barbara is constantly finding new ways to cope with her headaches.

If you are bothered by headaches as a result of MTBI, you have plenty of company! Headaches, from the mildly uncomfortable to the simply agonizing, are among the most common physical complaints following trauma to the head or neck. In this chapter, we will look at the various types of post-MTBI headaches, their causes, and conventional and alternative approaches to relieving headache pain. Also included are practical tips for minimizing or controlling headaches.

WHY HEADACHES CAN OCCUR AFTER MTBI

A single individual may experience headaches that range in intensity from mild to severe, and in quality from dull to sharp. The type of pain you experience depends on its point of origin. It can be experienced as a pounding, squeezing, tingling, or burning sensation; a touch-sensitive soreness; or a piercing jab that lasts anywhere from a second to several days.

Some headaches feel as though they originate deep within the skull; others seem to start externally and penetrate to the brain's very core. However, while it is the brain that perceives the discomfort of a headache, the brain itself is actually impervious to pain. What causes the experience of headache pain are pain sensors located in the arteries, nerves, and muscles of the head, as well as in the meninges (the thin membranes covering the brain), that have become distended, inflamed, or compressed.

TYPES OF HEADACHES THAT CAN FOLLOW MTBI

"During my recovery, I have experienced two types of headaches. Days after my accident, an excruciating neuralgic headache appeared. It felt as if someone were putting a hot poker into my skull. This intense pain went away after two months of anti-inflammatory medication prescribed by my neurologist. The other type of headache presented itself as a varied collection of symptoms that included an aura of lights or a distortion of perception, followed by neurological symptoms of facial numbness, severe right-side weakness, slurred speech, and thinking problems. My neurologist thought that these problems stemmed from partial seizures and prescribed anticonvulsant medication, which triggered numerous side effects, including dizziness. I was subsequently reevaluated by another doctor and diagnosed as suffering from posttraumic atypical migraines."

—D.R.S.

Medical researchers have identified more than a dozen different kinds of headaches. Of these, five are associated with MTBI: tension, migraine, posttraumatic, cluster, and analgesic-rebound. Each of these types of headaches has its own characteristics and causes.

It can be difficult to diagnose headaches precisely, however. After an MTBI, a phenomenon known as *symptom overlap* can occur. This happens when two or even three pain sources have been activated by injury, and it means that you may experience more than one kind of headache at a time, or you may alternate between different types of head pain depending on such factors as your activity level or the time of day. In addition, emotional stress, tension, or other physical pain can often increase headache pain.

Headaches come in many types and affect people differently. Even the dullest head pain can be incapacitating under certain circumstances. For the sake of clarity, we will look at each type of headache individually.

Tension Headache

If you suffer from tension headaches, you are already no doubt quite familiar with the two-sided sensation of squeezing or pressure that feels like a too-tight band around your head. The tightness continues for the duration of the headache, and may be accompanied by facial or back pain, particularly if you had a whiplash injury.

Tension headaches can be caused by worry, stress, poor posture, overwork, or inadequate ventilation. They often start late in the day, and they may prevent you from falling asleep. The pain may fluctuate from mild to moderate in intensity, but normal activity may not be affected. This is because physical activity does not generally aggravate tension headaches (in some cases, it may actually help).

Tension headaches are often described as either episodic or chronic. They are considered episodic if they occur fewer than fifteen times per month. Chronic tension headaches can persist for anywhere from fifteen days to six months at a time. These are often associated with depression—a common occurrence after MTBI. However, most tension headaches that follow MTBI stem from sudden injury to the vertebrae, muscles, ligaments, and tendons in the neck; or from an altered bite caused by damage to the teeth or injury to the temporomandibular (jaw) joint. Whichever of these is the case, the initial injury causes muscle spasms and inflamed, injured tissues, which in turn causes the pain.

Migraine Headache

Migraine headaches last from four to seventy-two hours and are experienced as an aching, pulsating, throbbing sensation at the forehead or temple. They may affect only one side of the head, or generalized areas of the skull. The physical effects may vary from one attack to the next or even within a single episode, and can include nausea and vomiting, muscle weakness, numbness, phonophobia (abnormal sensitivty to noise), photophobia (abnormal sensitivity to light), and osmophobia (abnormal sensitivity to smell). Migraines are typically intensified by physical activity and are often relieved by sleep.

Sometimes, migraines are preceded or accompanied by a set of sensory symptoms called an *aura*. An aura can include the perception of sudden brightness, jagged flashing lights, and/or blurred vision, and may also trigger problems with numbness, initiating movement, word-finding, speech, thinking and reasoning, and disorientation. Most auras occur twenty to sixty minutes prior to the onset of headache pain and last for twenty minutes or less.

Migraines are classified according to the extent that sensory symptoms are involved. If head pain is the only symptom, the condition is called *common migraine* or *migraine without aura*. If the head pain is preceded or accompanied by sensory symptoms, it is called a *classic migraine* or *migraine with aura*.

It is also possible to have the sensory symptoms of migraine—the aura—without the head pain. *Migraine equivalent,* or *painless migraine,* is characterized by an aura without a headache. Symptoms can include mood changes, dizziness, blurred vision, unexpected fatigue, and stomach discomfort. Another painless type occasionally seen is the *atypical migraine.* In this condition, along with the various symptoms present in an aura, other neurological symptoms may also be present, such as slurred speech and one-sided muscle weakness. This type of migraine is difficult to diagnose correctly because its symptoms are similar to those seen in mild stroke and in certain types of seizures. The relatively uncommon *basilar artery migraine (BAM)* involves a very intense aura and physical symptoms originating from either the brain stem or both occipital lobes (see Chapter 1). Typical BAM auras involve vision problems in both eyes, dizziness, loss of muscle coordination, speech problems, ringing in the ears, and a decrease in one's level of consciousness.

All types of migraines can be initiated by certain triggers. Common migraine triggers include such ordinary things as coughing, bending over, emotional stress, physical activity, the menstrual cycle, odors, sounds, and irregular eating or sleeping habits. Certain foods or combinations of foods can also lead to migraines (*see* Foods That Can Trigger or Worsen Headaches, page 63). Unusual fatigue, mood changes, bursts of energy, or excessive thirst or food cravings over a period of time can signal an impending migraine.

Posttraumatic Headache

This type of headache is associated with head trauma, and can arise months or even years after the original injury. A posttraumatic headache is not one specific type of headache, but rather can be a composite of a tension headache, atypical migraine, and neuralgic (nerve-related) head pain. The pain occurs when the formation of scar tissue, usually at the site of head trauma, renders the nerve-cell fibers

Foods That Can Trigger or Worsen Headaches

While not all headache sufferers are affected by what they eat, the consumption of certain foods can trigger headaches in some people. This is particularly true of people who suffer from migraines. Some of the most common headache-triggering foods and food ingredients include the following:

- *Alcohol*

- *Avocados*

- *Bananas*

- *Beans (except green or wax)*

- *Cheeses (ripened types, such as Cheddar or Brie)*

- *Chicken liver*

- *Chocolate*

- *Cured meats (such as bacon, bologna, or ham)*

- *Fermented, pickled, or marinated foods*

- *Figs (canned)*

- *Monosodium glutamate (MSG)*

- *Nuts*

- *Onions*

- *Peanut butter*

- *Peas*

- *Pizza*

- *Sour cream*

- *Vinegar (except white)*

- *Yeast-raised breads and cakes*

- *Yogurt*

If you are troubled by frequent headaches, you may be able to isolate a food culprit or two by eliminating all suspect items from your diet and seeing if your headaches improve. Then add back one food at a time to see which, if any, trigger headaches.

there unable to transmit information in the normal fashion. This disruption of impulses can cause the area of injury to become extremely sensitive, in a manner sometimes compared to that of the "funny bone" behind your elbow. The neuralgic component of this type of headache causes a burning or tingling sensation that radiates from the point of injury. The discomfort increases if any pressure is placed on the area, even pressure as light as a fingertip-touch or a gentle combing. The pain can be continuous, but, fortunately, most such headaches disappear within a year.

Cluster Headache

Cluster headaches are thought to be related to migraines. These severe headaches occur occasionally after MTBI, usually if injury to the back of the neck causes nerve damage and shooting pain or muscle spasms. A typical cluster headache appears suddenly and without warning, generally at a specific time of day, such as an hour or two after you fall asleep. The pain is an intense, steady, burning, penetrating sensation centered around or behind the eye and affecting only one side of the face. The involved eye may droop, tear, or become bloodshot; the cheek may be flushed; and the nostril on the affected side may be stuffy or runny. During an attack, symptoms may fluctuate from one side of the head to the other.

Cluster headache pain is quite severe and generally lasts from fifteen minutes to three hours. After that, discomfort may return in "clusters" of one to three headaches per day. Sometimes cluster-headache episodes alternate with periods of remission, but in some 20 percent of cases, the pain is chronic—occurring daily for a year or more. These headaches can be triggered by cigarette smoking, alcohol consumption, extreme emotion, overwork, or even unaccustomed relaxation.

Analgesic-Rebound Headache

This type of headache is a reaction to withdrawal from prolonged or excessive use of analgesics or ergot derivatives, which are drugs prescribed for pain relief. The pain may be severe and generalized across the head. Ironically, it is often more intense than the headache for which the medication was taken in the first place. The head pain may be accompanied by restlessness, irritability, nausea, difficulty concentrating, and feelings of depression. Some sufferers have difficulty falling asleep or staying asleep, or may be awakened very early by new head pain. Analgesic-rebound headaches can occur daily for as long as the problem medication is used, and can continue for several weeks beyond that until the offending drug is completely out of your system.

DIAGNOSING HEADACHES

A headache profile is one of the best ways to document your symptoms. This includes a preinjury headache history (many people's preinjury headaches were very different from those after the injury), a description of what the pain feels like, possible triggers, information about the pain's location and duration, and your thoughts on what seems to help. While headaches can have numerous symptoms and causes, and cover a broad spectrum of intensity, the acute symptoms are all treatable. Optimally, your head pain will subside completely once the right approach is found, but failing that, there are many ways to make any lingering discomfort quite manageable while you wait out the recovery process.

You will always have greater success nipping a headache in the bud than trying to end a full-blown episode. The key to doing this lies in correctly linking the headache's characteristics to its source, which in turn determines an initial course of pain relief. This is no easy task, however, since headaches can be difficult to identify and their causes hard to pin down. Also, different people react to pain differently, often according to their background and upbringing. Experiments with biofeedback have shown that the same bodily sensation that is called "uncomfortable" by one person may be termed "intolerable" by another. In addition, headache symptoms sometimes mimic other problems, including eyestrain, temporomandibular joint disorder, and seizure disorder. Moreover, as mentioned earlier, an MTBI can spawn more than one kind of headache, with symptom overlap that further complicates the issue.

It is therefore vital that you have professional input into your case, preferably with a treatment team that includes a neurologist who specializes in headaches. Depending on the location and circumstances of your injury, you may also benefit from the services of an orthopedist (a physician who specializes in disorders of the musculoskeletal system), a dentist, an ophthalmologist, an otolaryngologist, a physical therapist, and/or a psychologist. Together, you will have the best chance of understanding and eliminating the conditions that trigger your headache pain.

TREATING MTBI-RELATED HEADACHES

In general, headaches stop when the conditions that cause them are eliminated. Accomplishing this may be no small task when MTBI is involved, but there are a number of approaches, both conventional and alternative, that can act as preventive measures, and others that offer temporary pain relief when a headache occurs.

Conventional Approaches

"Since my MTBI, I suffer from occasional migraine headaches. After discovering that I had developed extreme sensitivity to prescription medication as a result of my MTBI, I found taking the homeopathic remedy Natrum muriaticum, *combined with EEG biofeedback, to be extremely effective for this type*

of pain. If I occasionally have a migraine without head pain, my neurologist suggested taking both acetaminophen and ibuprofen, and this seems to work."
—*D.R.S.*

Over-the-counter painkillers are the ideal starting place for anyone suffering from headaches, and they often bring relief to people with MTBI, many of whom find themselves newly responsive to low doses of medication. Well-known examples of these drugs include acetaminophen (Tylenol, Datril, and others), aspirin (Bayer, Bufferin, Ecotrin, and others); ibuprofen (Advil, Motrin, Nuprin, and others); ketoprofen (Actron and Orudis); and naproxen sodium (Aleve). There are also over-the-counter pain products that are combinations of aspirin and caffeine (Anacin) or acetaminophen and caffeine (Excedrin).

Each group of painkillers has specific advantages and particular side effects. The most appropriate way to select medication or a combination of medications is to weigh the different side effects and decide which are most endurable. Because your body can develop a tolerance to a single product, you can increase the effectiveness of over-the-counter drugs by varying the types you take—say, alternating between acetaminophen and ibuprofen. It is important to be cautious about doses, since analgesic-rebound headaches are a possibility with any pain medication.

Severe or persistent head pain may call for prescription medications. Many of these were initially developed for other maladies but can also be effective against headaches. For instance, certain drugs used for cardiovascular problems, particularly beta-blockers and calcium-channel blockers, reduce pain because they interfere with the transmission of nerve impulses in the circulatory and respiratory systems, thus keeping the blood vessels in the head from becoming constricted. Other types of drugs, including some antihistamines, anticonvulsants (anti-seizure medications), ergot derivatives, antidepressants, and even steroids can also block the pain of certain types of headaches by reducing inflammation, relaxing muscles, or disrupting nerve activity in key areas of the body. (*See* Drugs Used for Headaches, page 67, for a list of medications commonly used to prevent and treat headaches related to MTBI.)

Your choice of headache medication will depend on several factors: the nature of your MTBI; the type and intensity of resulting pain; your medical history and the other medications you take; and the results you have experienced with other headache remedies. Your health-care provider should tailor his or her recommendations to your particular circumstances and monitor your usage carefully. Diagnostic

Drugs Used for Headaches

There are many different medications that have helped people who suffer from headaches following MTBI. Some of these are used to relieve headache pain; others are more useful as preventives. The following table lists some of the types of drugs most commonly used for headaches, plus examples of each type. For each drug listed, the generic name is given first, followed by the brand name or names in parentheses.

Type of Drug	Use	Examples
Analgesics	General pain relief and headache prevention	Aspirin (Bayer, Bufferin Ecotrin, and others) Acetaminophen (Tylenol, Datril, and others) Combinations (Anacin, Excedrin, Fiorinal Medigesic, and others)
Anticonvulsants	Headache prevention; also used to control seizure activity	Phenytoin (Dilantin) Valproic acid (Depakene)
Antidepressants	Pain relief and headache prevention; also used for treament of depression	Amitriptyline (Elavil, Endep) Doxepin (Adapin, Sinequan) Fluoxetine (Prozac) Nortriptyline (Aventyl, Pamelor) Phenelzine (Nardil)
Antihistamines	Headache prevention; also used for treatment of allergy symptoms	Cyproheptadine (Periactin)
Beta-blockers	Headache prevention; also used for treatment of high blood pressure and heart problems	Atenolol (Tenormin) Nadolol (Corgard) Propranolol (Inderal) Timolol (Blocadren)
Calcium-channel blockers	Headache prevention; also used for treatment of high blood pressure	Diltiazem (Cardizem) Nifedipine (Adalat, Procardia) Nimodipine (Nimotop) Verapamil (Calan, Isoptin)

Type of Drug	Use	Examples
Ergot derivatives	Pain relief and headache prevention, especially for migraine and cluster headaches	Dihydroergotamine (D.H.E. 45) Ergotamine (Ergostat) Ergotamine combinations (Bellergal-S [also contains phenobarbital, belladonna alkaloids], Cafergot [also contains caffeine]) Methylergonovine (Methergine) Methysergide (Sansert)
Narcotics	Treatment of intense, persistent pain	Meperidine (Demerol) Oxycodone combinations (Percocet, Roxicet, Tylox [also contain acetaminophen], Percodan [also contains aspirin])
Nonsteroidal anti-inflammatories (NSAIDs)	General pain relief and headache prevention	Ibuprofen (Advil, Motrin, Nuprin, and others) Indomethacin (Indocin) Ketoprofen (Actron, Orudis) Naproxen (Naprosyn) Naproxen sodium (Aleve, Anaprox)
Steroids	Treatment of intense, persistent pain	Dexamethasone (Decadron, Hexadrol, and others) Prednisone (Deltasone, Sterapred, and others)
Tranquilizers	Treatment of intense, persistent pain	Chlorpromazine (Thorazine) Haloperidol (Haldol) Thiothixene (Navane)

Not all drugs help all individuals. It may be necessary for your doctor to try several different prescriptions before finding the one that works best for you. It should be noted that sumatriptan (Imitrex), one of the newer drugs used to treat acute migraine episodes, is generally not recommended for people who have suffered MTBI.

tests and a trial-and-error approach may be necessary to find the most effective medication for you.

It is important to stress that not every medication is effective for every person. In addition, like almost all medications, headache drugs have numerous potential side effects, ranging from stomach upset to blurred vision, from dizziness to slowed heart rate. Some drugs can worsen preexisting health problems or have serious, even deadly, side effects if taken in improper doses. If you are taking medication for headaches, following your doctor's usage instructions carefully can mean the difference between pain relief and permanent problems.

Another approach that may be helpful for headaches is psychotherapy. Psychotherapy can help to pinpoint and alleviate depression, which can precede or accompany chronic headaches. Behavioral medicine, a branch of psychotherapy that includes such techniques as biofeedback, hypnosis, cognitive-behavioral therapy, and relaxation training, has been helpful for some people with MTBI. Extensive research has shown that biofeedback done by a licensed clinical psychophysiologist can be very effective against chronic headache pain. One downside of this type of treatment, however, is that the numerous sessions that may be required can become costly if not covered by insurance.

Hypnosis is similar to biofeedback in that it can help you learn to control bodily sensations. While biofeedback uses mechanical devices to do this, with hypnosis you learn to monitor your body through intense focusing, initially with the aid of a health psychologist and then on your own. Pain-control techniques for chronic headaches may involve visualizing a cold compress on your forehead or an on/off "pain switch" similar to a light switch. With instruction and a bit of practice, even children can become adept at this practice. However, the effective use of hypnosis does require concentration, which is often a problem after MTBI.

Cognitive-behavioral therapy is often combined with biofeedback and/or hypnosis. This type of therapy involves exploring the connection between cognition (thoughts), beliefs, feelings, behavior, and pain. A licensed psychologist who is board certified in behavioral or health psychology can provide tools for coping with the lifestyle repercussions of long-term pain, as well as strategies for managing stress and other conditions that contribute to headaches.

Developing a relaxation response is a good way to reduce stress, release tensed muscles, and combat hormonal changes that can result in headaches. Proficiency at yoga, meditation, visualization, and other relaxation techniques, such as those described in Herbert Benson's *The Relaxation Response* (Avon, 1976), can give you a natural defense against pain. The degree of relaxation needed to minimize pain varies from person to person and according to the specific type of headache.

The relaxation response is easy to practice. You need ten to twenty minutes of free time—perhaps before breakfast—and should arrange not to be disturbed. Find a place where you are comfortable, close your eyes, and relax your muscles. Breathe slowly in through your nose and out through your mouth while repeating and focusing on a word or phrase. When you finish, sit quietly for a minute or two— first with your eyes closed, then with them opened.

The hands-on techniques of physical therapy, including massage and stretching exercises, can be effective against headaches associated with muscle spasms and pain in the face and neck. Water therapy and ultrasound techniques are similarly helpful. Other methods some people use to control headache pain include aerobic exercise such as brisk walking or swimming; maintaining consistent sleep patterns; and dietary monitoring to avoid trigger foods (see page 63). If you smoke, quitting may help. For the most stubborn pain, headache clinics and pain clinics can teach additional methods of controlling your discomfort.

Alternative Approaches

While medication is likely to be an element in the treatment of MTBI-related headaches, there is also much to be said for other approaches to pain relief. Nondrug treatments, which are far less risky than drug therapy, may reduce the frequency and intensity of your headaches. Even if a nondrug approach to headache pain is not completely effective by itself, it can often reduce your need for medication. It is advisable, therefore, to consider and experiment with other approaches to headache pain—under your doctor's supervision, of course.

Chiropractic treatment has been shown to be effective in treating posttraumatic, tension-type, and some migraine headaches. Chiropractic manipulation by a licensed chiropractor reduces abnormal motion and irritation to the neck muscles, nerves, and other tissues.

Acupuncture helps control headache pain by stimulating the release of endorphins, body chemicals that act as natural pain relievers. After an initial evaluation, an acupuncturist inserts hairlike needles into specific points on your body. A session usually lasts thirty to fifty minutes. While improvement generally begins in twenty minutes, subsequent sesions are usually needed to control chronic headaches. A related type of treatment, acupressure, can be effective at the onset of headache pain. This involves pressing and then rotating the fingertips firmly against certain points on the body, such as the temples, the top of the head, the hollows in front of the jaw muscles, or below the bones at the base of the skull. The appropriate points depend on the nature and location of your headaches. It is best to consult with a licensed acupuncturist to determine your specific acupressure needs.

You may also want to consider using homeopathic remedies and herbal preparations for headaches. Herbs such as arnica, feverfew, peppermint, skullcap, and white willow bark have long been used to relieve headache pain, and feverfew is in fact approved as a migraine treatment by many neurologists. Relaxing herbs such as chamomile may be helpful as well. Homeopathic remedies that may be recommended for headaches include *Bryonia, Ferrum phosphoricum, Gelsemium,* and *Natrum muriaticum.* There are also homeopathic combination remedies available for headaches. As with all homeopathic treatment, the appropriate remedy depends on the precise nature of the symptoms. Both herbal and homeopathic remedies should be treated with the same respect as any other type of medicine. It is wise to consult a professional herbalist or homeopath who has experience in treating MTBI to ensure that over-the-counter herbs and homeopathic remedies are right for you.

PRACTICAL SUGGESTIONS

Controlling headache discomfort can be a formidable task. A good place to start is with identifying and eliminating environmental factors that seem to bring on head pain. There isn't always a single headache trigger, of course, but you can cultivate habits to counteract factors that often lead to headaches. You can also take action to stop a developing headache before it takes hold. The following are practical suggestions that can help:

- Schedule time—even if just ten minutes a day—to learn how to relax. Find a pleasant location, wear loose clothing, and practice simple visualization or deep breathing.

- Document each headache episode. Each time a headache strikes, record the date, the time of day, foods eaten recently, your emotions and activity level around the time of the attack, and anything else that may be relevant. Then try to modify your environment to eliminate potential headache causes.

- Eliminate from your diet any foods that have been shown to trigger headaches. If you are not sure which foods may be involved, start by eliminating the most common offenders (*see* Foods That Can Trigger or Worsen Headaches on page 63).

- Try not to deviate from your normal sleeping, exercise, and meal-time schedule.

- Try to determine whether certain activities—say, bending over, drinking alcohol, or squinting—seem to trigger headaches. Then avoid suspect activities as much as possible.

- Increase your level of aerobic fitness (but stick to low-impact exercises such as swimming or walking).

- Be aware that weather conditions, such as high humidity and the drop in barometric pressure that often precedes a summer storm, can contribute to migraines. It is advisable to monitor the weather as well as to experiment with controllable triggers.

- Avoid fluorescent lighting, if possible. This and other types of pulsating light cause stress on the eyes as well as mental strain.

- At the first sign of a tension headache, apply heat to your forehead and temples using warmed hands or a dampened face cloth. If heat brings no relief, try placing a cold gel-pack or ice pack on your forehead or the top of your head.

- At the first sign of a migraine headache, change your surroundings for a relaxing setting. If possible, lie down and sleep.

- At the first sign of a neuralgic heachache, lightly brush or comb your scalp. This may help to minimize head pain.

There is no question that chronic headaches leave their mark on all aspects of your life. Remember that your MTBI has made you somewhat fragile. It is acceptable—even advisable—to pamper yourself physically throughout the healing process and to make avoiding stress a new priority in your life. Patience, a positive attitude, your doctor's guidance, and the understanding of your family and friends are the tools that will best help you to minimize and cope with your discomfort.

6

DIZZINESS

New Yorker Mary Beth is the survivor of two MTBIs—the second one eight years after the first, and both from skiing accidents. It was the second injury that really affected her. Someone skied into her at the bottom of a slope, striking her head, injuring her back, and knocking her jaw out of place. It took the ski patrol over forty-five minutes to come to Mary Beth's aid, and when she was transported to the hospital, the emergency-room physician made several poor judgments. Mary Beth said that every time she moved or reclined, the room seemed to spin—it felt as if she were on a carnival ride. The doctor dismissed this, saying that it was just a result of lying down too long, and the only thing he did was to order a back x-ray.

Mary Beth was a program research specialist with the New York State Department of Health and an adjunct instructor at a community college. She continued to teach her classes after the second accident, but her dizziness kept her from driving and caused her to feel that the room was spinning whenever she turned from the chalkboard to look out into the lecture hall.

After her second MTBI, a neurologist told Mary Beth that she was "as normal as normal could be." Fortunately, her long-time family physician saw the change in her and helped her to seek the treatment she needed. She is now seeing a neuropsychologist and a psychiatrist to help her put her life back together. Her classroom dizziness has now stopped and Mary Beth can drive again. However, she still experiences occasional lightheadedness when she gets up too quickly—a feeling that she, rather than the room, is spinning.

At one time or another, virtually everyone—MTBI survivor or not—experiences the unsettling sensation of dizziness. The room seems to spin, your vision dims momentarily, and you become aware of a slightly nauseated feeling. Dizziness can be related to several conditions, among them low blood sugar, extreme hunger, and low blood pressure.

WHY DIZZINESS CAN OCCUR AFTER MTBI

Dizziness is a common complaint after traumatic brain injury, and there are a number of reasons for the symptom. Double vision, injury to brain stem centers that monitor balance, or damage to certain areas of your cerebellum can trigger lightheadedness or a feeling of imbalance. Blood pressure fluctuations, caused by disruption of the nerve impulses that govern your heart rate or by trauma to the part of the brain that regulates blood flow, can also make you feel faint or unsteady. Extended use of a cervical collar, a supportive device for the neck that is often recommended after a whiplash injury, can lead to compression of nerves leading into the back of the head and, in turn, increased lightheadedness. Vertigo is usually caused by injury to an inner-ear structure called the semicircular canal.

WHAT MTBI-RELATED DIZZINESS IS LIKE

"After my MTBI, I had problems with feeling lightheaded, unbalanced, and unsteady. In one situation, I was on a small rowboat for an hour and couldn't regain a feeling of steadiness for more than three hours after returning to land. Many of my medications increased these feelings, especially the products taken to combat high blood pressure and seizures."

—D.R.S.

There is a difference between dizziness—feeling lightheaded and unsteady—and the sensation called vertigo. If the dizziness you experience is true vertigo, you will feel that the room is spinning around you whenever your head or body moves into certain positions, particularly if the change in position is rapid. Research shows that from 15 to 78 percent of people with MTBI experience vertigo as a consequence of their injuries.

If your dizziness stems from lightheadedness or an unbalanced feeling, you will not feel that your surroundings are spinning, but as if *you* are spinning. You may need to hold onto a chair or tabletop because your sense of where you are in the room seems so fleeting. The feeling of not having your "sea legs" may be constantly with you. You may find yourself avoiding unnecessary movement so that you won't trigger yet another unpleasant wave of disequilibrium—particularly in the morning hours, when unsteadiness is usually at its peak.

DIAGNOSING DIZZINESS

To distinguish between MTBI-induced vertigo and lightheadedness that may be caused by another problem, your doctor should take a medical history and check your blood pressure in a sitting or standing position. If your blood pressure is normal and your symptoms may be from true vertigo, your physician will likely refer you to one or more of the following specialists: an otolaryngologist, an ophthalmologist, a neurologist, and/or an endocrinologist. These specialists can determine whether your dizziness symptoms stem from inner-ear, vision, central nervous system, or endocrine system disorders.

Evaluating inner-ear function is important for distinguishing between true vertigo and other types of balance problems, which in turn is essential to formulating an appropriate treatment plan. Two important tests that may be done by a neuro-otolaryngologist to evaluate your vestibular system (the balance system in your inner ear) are the *caloric test* and the *rotary chair test*. In the caloric test, your inner ear is alternately cooled and heated by irrigation with water at controlled temperatures, while your eye movements are monitored by means of an instrument called an electronystagmograph. Because the body normally responds to such temperature stimulation with characteristic movements of the eyeball, this test can diagnose problems in the vestibular system. In the rotary chair test, your eye movements are measured as you focus on a fixed object while sitting in a slowly turning chair.

TREATING MTBI-RELATED DIZZINESS

Fortunately, dizziness or vertigo that results from an MTBI usually subsides within six to eight weeks. However, those long days of discomfort can seem interminable, particularly if the dizziness makes you feel nauseated or you are struggling to deal with other aftereffects of your injury. There are a number of approaches you can try to minimize your episodes of dizziness—or better still, to bring the entire malady to a quicker end. These can be used either by themselves or in conjunction with other approaches.

Conventional Approaches

Occasionally, vertigo can be so severe that it renders you unable to function. If this happens, an over-the-counter motion sickness product such as dimenhydrinate (Dramamine), cyclizine (Marezine), or a prescription medication for dizziness and nausea such as meclizine (Antivert; also available in nonprescription strength as Bonine) can bring

relief. Vertigo can sometimes be minimized through the use of seda-
tives such as diazepam (Valium). Another helpful approach is physical therapy with a practitioner who specializes in balance and spatial-
orientation problems. Not every therapist is trained to treat MTBIs
and dizziness. However, the right person can teach you exercises that
temporarily overload the vestibular system. Overloading challenges the
vestibular system to adapt to multiple atypical movements. For example, you may be asked to sit or lie atop a large ball and move
your arms or legs in specific patterns. A similar type of approach is
used by figure skaters, who practice spinning and twirling until they
can perform such moves without dizziness.

Alternative Approaches

Acupressure can help an attack of dizziness to abate. When dizziness
strikes, try applying steady, firm pressure to your temples and to your
jaw joints, directly in front of your ears, for several minutes or until
dizziness subsides. Auricular, or outer ear, acupuncture has also been
shown to be helpful in relieving dizziness, as well as in heading off
future episodes. Chiropractic treatment may also help.

There are several herbs and homeopathic remedies that can combat dizziness problems as well. However, since dizziness that is related to MTBI may be only one of your symptoms, you should consult with a qualified herbalist or homeopath about what is best for
you rather than experimenting on your own with over-the-counter
preparations. The Herb Research Foundation and/or the National Center for Homeopathy (see the Resources section beginning on page 281)
can be of assistance in locating an experienced practitioner in your
area.

PRACTICAL SUGGESTIONS

*"I've learned to cope with attacks of dizziness by casually leaning on a wall
or gently touching a desk. When walking, I look for a straight-line focal point,
like the grout line between floor tiles."*

—*Julia*

While it is always a good idea to seek professional assistance with a
symptom as problematic as dizziness, you can do a lot at home and
work to keep attacks at bay, or at least to lessen their severity. Here
are a number of ideas:

• At the first sign of dizziness, stop moving and sit or lie down. In
  most instances, this helps the sensation to pass within a few minutes.

- Roll out of bed slowly in the morning rather than quickly sitting upright.

- Modify your activities and environment so that you either avoid or bombard your system with dizziness triggers. For example, either sit and stand up slowly, so as not to set off the motion receptors in your inner ear, or try repeating these movements in rapid succession until the accompanying spinning sensation stops.

- Note whether your dizziness is worse at certain times of day, when you are hungry, or if you spend time amid warm temperatures, bright sunlight, or noise. If it is, take steps to avoid these conditions.

- Try sleeping without a pillow so that your neck and upper spine remain perfectly straight and your head is not pushed forward while you sleep. A folded hand towel or piece of fabric tucked under or behind the neck can increase your comfort in this position. Special cervical pillows, available in many drugstores, also offer gentle support for the neck.

- Use support such as a cervical collar—under a doctor's supervision, of course—if you have suffered a neck or whiplash injury. Doing so temporarily can take pressure off crucial nerves in the area.

- Be aware that drugs such as oral contraceptives and blood pressure medications can cause dizziness as a side effect. In fact, some medication-sensitive individuals may even get dizzy after taking aspirin. Bear in mind that your MTBI may have made you more sensitive than normal to medication. Be sure to confer with your doctor before taking any drug product.

- Avoid alcohol, cigarettes, and recreational drugs, since these substances promote dizziness.

- Limit your use of salt, which can cause fluid retention and increased vertigo.

Dizziness is one of the more vague symptoms of MTBI because it can be triggered by several different conditions. Happily, though, it is likely to be one of your shorter-lived complaints. While you wait for the unpleasant sensation to subside, it is worthwhile to experiment with different methods of making yourself more comfortable. With time, patience, and the right techniques, your dizziness should soon be a thing of the past.

7

SEXUALITY

Beverley, a successful real-estate broker and nationally rated gymnastics judge, had been happily married for thirty-two years. Prior to her brain injury, she often initiated lovemaking with her husband, whether by preparing a candlelit dinner, wearing an alluring nightgown, or just engaging in provocative play. After her MTBI, she felt as if sexuality did not exist. Sex never entered her mind, she never felt aroused, and the idea of initiating sexual intimacy was completely foreign to her. It took almost two years before Beverley began to make overtures toward lovemaking, and even then, it took a very conscious effort.

You may have found your sexual side to be curiously absent in the time since your MTBI. Or perhaps the opposite is true—since your injury, you may have found yourself consumed with thoughts of sex and the desire for intimate physical contact. In either case, you may be relieved to know that this is no mere coincidence. While sexual issues are rarely granted the attention paid to other MTBI symptoms, there is a sound basis for these problems.

WHY SEXUAL PROBLEMS CAN OCCUR AFTER MTBI

Contrary to popular belief, the state of sexual arousal has its roots in the brain, not in the sex organs or erogenous zones. Just as your brain signals the need for nourishment or sleep, it also determines when—and if—you become sexually aroused. Specifically, the desire for sex is regulated by the hypothalamus, as well as the brain stem and surrounding structures (see Chapter 1).

If your MTBI is localized in this area, your brain may be unable to properly receive, interpret, or relay information transmitted by other parts of the body. Thus, what seems like a sudden loss of sexual drive is actually a neurological malfunction that blocks pleasurable images, thoughts, and sensations. Less commonly, a force or blow to the brain's frontal lobe causes sudden problems in the ability to reason, make judgments, and conduct yourself in a socially appropriate manner. One result of such an injury can be a sharp, even problematic, increase in sexual desire and activity.

Sexual difficulties can also stem from concentration problems (problems with concentration will be discussed in detail in Chapter 13). The extent to which you can relax and enjoy physical contact is directly related to your capacity to screen out distractions. Loss of the ability to focus in this manner can make it difficult, if not impossible, to become and remain aroused. Chronic pain, sleep deprivation, and emotional upheaval—also common occurrences after MTBI—can have similar effects on sexual desire. In addition, prescription medications that are used to treat postinjury headaches, seizures, and other symptoms may dull sexual response by interfering with nervous system signals that accompany arousal. Most antidepressants are similarly troublesome in that they alter brain chemicals, including those that determine desire, sensation, and climax time.

SEXUAL PROBLEMS THAT CAN FOLLOW MTBI

"My accident took place in March, and I thought that by November, my life would be like it used to be—including a normal sex life. I had a healthy, active sexual response prior to my MTBI, but for eight months after, my sex life with my husband came to a halt. I had no desire and was sexually numb and unresponsive. Extrememly concerned, I asked my neurologist about this. His response was, "This can happen with a head injury. The problem you're experiencing might also be caused by your medication." I wanted to scream. No one had ever told me that this could happen because of a head injury!"
—*D.R.S.*

A normal, active sexual relationship has interrelated physical, mental, and psychological components. Understandably, a problem with even one facet can have a significant effect on the quality of the relationship as a whole. If you are still having sexual problems that are unrelated to medication six months after your MTBI, you can assume that the problems are a direct result of brain trauma. If you had sexual problems prior to your injury, your symptoms may intensify. What follows is a look at the various sexual difficulties that can occur as a result of MTBI.

Loss of Desire

Whether your MTBI or subsequent medication has interrupted the transmission of pleasure signals, left you unable to concentrate, or triggered pain, worry, or sleeplessness, you are likely to experience diminished sexual drive. In light of the strain of your injury and the energy you are devoting to recovery, sex may start seeming unimportant or just like more trouble than it's worth.

Altered Sensation

If the brain's pleasure center fails to interpret incoming nerve impulses properly, sexual contact can fail to have its customary arousing effect. Instead, normally erogenous areas of the body may seem deadened and disconnected from the arousal process. In other cases, the breasts, genitals, and other sexual areas may become unbearably sensitive, so that sexual touch feels annoying or uncomfortable.

Physiological Problems

In the absense of brain signals of arousal—or in spite of them, where certain medications are concerned—physiological changes that normally precede intercourse may fail to occur in the usual fashion. For men, this can mean an inability to achieve or sustain an erection due to diminished blood flow to the penis. A woman may be unable to lubricate or relax the vaginal muscles. Many different medications, some of which are often prescribed for MTBI-related symptoms, can interfere with normal sexual functioning. In addition, anyone who has suffered an MTBI may be rendered more sensitive to medications in general, whether taken for MTBI-related problems or not, even if these drugs previously caused no adverse effects. Table 7.1 gives examples of medications often prescribed for people with MTBI that can cause sexual dysfunction as a side effect.

Intensified Sexual Desire

While a significantly heightened sexual drive is usually associated with moderate and severe brain injuries, this condition occasionally occurs as a result of MTBI. In some cases, this intensified drive is manageable. In other instances, it can become overwhelming and compel an individual to make inappropriate jokes, comments, and physical advances, or to engage in exhibitionism and other overtly sexual behavior in public.

Table 7.1 Drugs That Can Cause Sexual Dysfunction

Medication	Possible Sexual Effects
ANTIANXIETY AGENTS	
Diazepam (Valium)	Reduced sexual desire; impotence; inhibited orgasm; inhibited ejaculation
Lorazepam (Ativan)	Loss of desire
ANTICONVULSANTS	
Carbamazepine (Atretol, Tegretol)	Impotence
Ethosuximide (Zarontin)	Increased sexual desire
Phenytoin (Dilantin)	Reduced sexual desire; impotence; persistent, painful erections
Primidone (Mysoline)	Reduced sexual desire; impotence
ANTIDEPRESSANTS	
Amitriptyline (Elavil, Endep)	Loss of desire; impotence; inhibited ejaculation
Doxepin (Adapin, Sinequan)	Reduced sexual desire; inhibited ejaculation
Fluoxetine (Prozac)	Reduced sexual desire; inhibited orgasm; inhibited ejaculation; loss of penile sensation
Nortriptyline (Aventyl, Pamelor)	Reduced sexual desire; impotence
Phenelzine (Nardil)	Impotence; inhibited orgasm; inhibited ejaculation; persistent, painful erections
Sertraline (Zoloft)	Sexual dysfunction
BETA-BLOCKERS	
Atenolol (Tenormin)	Impotence
Labetalol (Normodyne, Trandate)	Reduced sexual desire; impotence; inhibited ejaculation; persistent, painful erections
Metoprolol (Lopressor)	Impotence
Propranolol (Inderal)	Loss of desire; impotence
Timolol (Blocadren)	Reduced sexual desire; impotence
CALCIUM-CHANNEL BLOCKERS	
Nifedipine (Adalat, Procardia)	Persistent, painful erections
Verapamil (Calan, Isoptin, Verelan)	Impotence

Medication	Possible Sexual Effects
PAIN MEDICATION/ANTI-INFLAMMATORIES	
Indomethacin (Indocin)	Reduced sexual desire; impotence
Naproxen (Naprosyn)	Impotence; inhibited ejaculation
Naproxen sodium (Aleve, Anaprox)	Impotence; inhibited ejaculation
TRANQUILIZERS	
Chlorpromazine (Thorazine)	Reduced sexual desire; impotence; inhibited ejaculation
Haloperidol (Haldol)	Impotence; pain upon ejaculation
Thiothixene (Navane)	Impotence; persistent, painful erections; spontaneous ejaculation
MISCELLANEOUS	
Acetazolamide (Diamox)	Loss of desire; impotence
Baclofen (Lioresal)	Impotence; inhibited ejaculation
Dextroamphetamine (Dexedrine)	Impotence; inhibited orgasm; inhibited ejaculation

Relationship Problems

Changes in desire or drive can trigger other problems in your relationship with your sexual partner. For example, if MTBI causes you to lose interest in sex, it is not unusual to fear that your partner will take offense or lose patience and seek sex elsewhere. A diminished sexual drive can also lead you to withhold affection, become less communicative, and otherwise avoid situations and behavior that might lead to intimate physical contact. Anxiety over your ability to perform or to enjoy sexual activity can compound sexual problems by adding an element of stress. A sudden increase in the sexual demands of one partner can cause stress in a relationship as well.

Unfortunately, we often do not see sexual problems as serious enough to need attention until they have lasted long enough to cause emotional or marital problems—in fact, it is usually these secondary problems that cause people to seek professional help.

DIAGNOSING SEXUAL PROBLEMS

If you are troubled by changes in your sexual drive or ability, it is important to volunteer the information promptly and candidly when your primary health-care provider asks the customary question, "How are you doing?" Understandably, most doctors rely on their patients to advise them of less-than-obvious symptoms and complaints. Since sex is a more personal topic than, say, dizziness or memory problems, few medical professionals probe this aspect of their patients' postconcussive symptoms. Some may be reluctant to address the issue even if it is raised by the patient. In addition, many doctors feel that warning people with MTBI about the possibility of sexual problems may cause unnecessary worry and anxiety—not all people are affected by this problem, and those who are may be affected for only a relatively short time. However, if you do experience sexual problems and these are not addressed, your physical and emotional symptoms can escalate.

When discussing sexual problems with your doctor, it is important to emphasize the way in which your current situation represents a change from the past. After all, the definition of "normal" sexual desire and performance varies greatly from individual to individual and from couple to couple. The fact that your sexual responsiveness differs from what it was before the injury is what is most important. You should also consider your other MTBI symptoms—insomnia or inattentiveness, for instance—and raise the possibility of a link between these symptoms (and medications you may take for them) and your newfound sexual difficulties.

Your doctor or practitioner will probably suggest an examination by a gynecologist or urologist to rule out physical dysfunction unrelated to your brain injury. He or she may also refer you to a mental health professional for emotional support and further consideration of your problem.

TREATING MTBI-RELATED SEXUAL PROBLEMS

Of all post-MTBI symptoms, sexual problems can be among the hardest to cope with. This is because it is often harder to obtain support from your partner, who is directly affected by the situation. Also, it can be difficult to discuss this topic with family and friends. Knowing this, you may be tempted to wait out your difficulties or let them go unattended while you focus on other aspects of recovery. However, it is critical to your state of mind—and quite possibly to your relationship with your partner—that you obtain the help you need to get your sexual side back on track. A number of approaches to resolving sexual problems are presented below. Additional information and support can be obtained from resources listed at the end of this book.

Conventional Approaches

If your sexual problems are medication related, time will not improve things. Discuss with your doctor the possibility of switching medications or modifying dosages to reverse, or at least minimize, sexual side effects.

Psychotherapy, including hypnosis and biofeedback, and behavioral sex therapy by a physician-recommended specialist can provide insight into sexual difficulties and often reignite—or, if necessary, temper—your libido. Couple counseling can also be extremely helpful for promoting mutual understanding of your problem and reducing tension between you and your partner. If your problem involves inappropriate sexual remarks or behavior, a rehabilitation or Veterans' Administration hospital (whether or not you are a veteran) can refer you to a professional with specialization in sexual disorders stemming from brain injury.

For women, if arousal is a problem, you might consider the use of an artificial lubricant such as K-Y jelly, and/or do Kegel exercises to tone the vaginal muscles. Both of these measures can make sexual stimulation and intercourse more pleasurable. Kegel exercises consist of tightening and squeezing the vagina and rectum by drawing the muscles inward and upward, holding this position for five to ten seconds, then relaxing. This can be done virtually anywhere, at any time. You should try to do at least thirty repetitions a day. In males for whom erectile problems or loss of sensations appear to be permanent, a urologist may recommend one of a number of approaches to reverse impotence (usually medication, a penile implant, or a vacuum device). For women, surgery to expose the clitoris or tighten the pubococcygeus muscle, in which are located the nerve endings responsible for sensation in the outer section of the vagina, may be an option.

Alternative Approaches

Certain herbal remedies, when used appropriately, can bolster libido or counteract the effects of medication on drive and performance. Damiana, sno yang, yin yan hyo, ba jitian, green oats, and wild yam, for instance, have long been considered to enhance sexuality when taken in balanced herbal preparations. *Ginko biloba* may be helpful in reversing medication-related impotence and loss of desire. It is best to consult with a qualified herbalist who has training and experience in treating people with head injuries and sexual dysfunction. Similarly, a homeopathic physician may be able to recommend appropriate remedies, as well as dietary changes and other natural measures, that can produce positive results. Homeopathic remedies often recommended for sexual problems include *Sepia, Silica, Natrum muriaticum,* and *Kali phosphoricum.*

PRACTICAL SUGGESTIONS

While it is crucial to seek professional help for sexual and other difficulties triggered by your MTBI, there are helpful measures that you can try on your own. The first and most important thing is to be forthright with your partner about the existence and nature of the changes in your sexual side. You may wish to consider and discuss the following suggestions:

- Try various methods of relaxation before engaging in sex, including a warm bath, massage, meditation, or deep-breathing exercises. Maintain your state of relaxation by allowing sufficient time for leisurely-paced sexual activity.

- Do what you can to block out distracting stimuli during sex. Lock the door, darken the room, warm the sheets with an electric blanket, and shut out noise with music or the drone of an electric fan.

- Consider props to increase arousal. The use of candles, body oil, soothing music, erotic apparel, and visual aids such as books or films can help you stay focused during sex.

- Consult the *Physician's Desk Reference (PDR)*, found in the reference section of most public libraries, for information about potential adverse reactions to any drugs you take, including such "ordinary" drugs as antihistamines, diuretics, and cholesterol medication. If "changed libido" or "genitourinary complaints" are listed as a possibility, ask your doctor whether you might stop the medication or switch to a different drug. *Do not,* however, discontinue any prescribed medication without consulting with your physician.

Above all, it is important not to minimize your sexual difficulties, and it is equally important not to blame yourself for them. Remember that in more than half of all cases, these problems have a physical cause, and that in fully 25 percent of such cases, sexual problems are directly related to medication.

While time may be the best healer for many MTBI-related problems, treatment is widely available for most types of sexual dysfunction. You will be best able to cope with sexual changes that are MTBI related if you communicate with and muster the support of your partner, and then arm yourself with knowledge about aspects of your injury that might be contributing to your problem. Having done that, you can continue consulting and working with appropriate professionals until you get the help you need.

8

VISION PROBLEMS

Patricia suffered an MTBI when her car was struck head-on at thirty-seven miles per hour by a truck that failed to yield the right of way. In the early stages of her recovery, Patricia often saw double images and had problems moving her eyes across the page when reading. She also had difficulty watching moving objects and tolerating bright and fluorescent lights.

These problems have improved over time, but Patricia still has days when she is extra-sensitive to visual stimulation. To cope with her sensitivity, she sometimes plays games, for instance, telling herself that this is one of those days when she has to keep her eyes from wandering to nonessential sights.

While you might not immediately connect an injury to your neck or a blow to the back of your head with the onset of vision problems, the fact is that a great many people who have suffered MTBIs experience trouble with their eyes. Double vision and blurred vision are the most common complaints, but a wide range of other maladies, including partial vision loss, tracking difficulties (problems focusing on moving objects), and photophobia (abnormal sensitivity to light) can also occur.

As with other MTBI symptoms, the extent and duration of vision problems depend on the force, type, and location of brain trauma. In some cases, a complete return to normal vision may be unlikely; however, many people with MTBI experience significant if not complete improvement over the long term. Regardless of your prognosis, it is important to understand the nature of the vision problems brought on by MTBI.

WHY VISION PROBLEMS CAN OCCUR AFTER MTBI

Vision is a complex process that involves not only the eyes but also the brain. Light enters the eye and is focused by the lens and projected onto the retina, where an image of whatever the eyes are looking at is formed. This image is then transmitted by means of the optic nerve to the occipital lobe, located at the back of the brain. This part of the brain houses the visual pathways that receive nerve impulses from the retina. It also controls your visual fields and your understanding of what you see. The process of seeing is made even more complex by the fact that, because of the way light enters the eye, the image that forms on the retina is reversed. That is, images of things to your right form on the left side of the retina, and vice versa. This image reversal is itself compensated for—the image is re-reversed—by the way in which nerve impulses from the retina travel to the brain. Images from the right side of the retina go to the right side of the brain, and those from the left side of the retina go to the left side of the brain (remember that the right side of the brain controls the left side of the body, and vice versa).

The eye and the optic nerve therefore constitute an intricate instrument that is vulnerable to a number of different injuries. Sometimes the eyeball itself sustains a direct blow during an MTBI. When this happens, the force of impact can bend, compress, twist, tear, or jolt the lens, the retina, and/or the optic nerve, all of which are critical to seeing correctly. In other instances, an impact injury to the base of the skull or the back of the neck may damage delicate tissues in the brain stem that regulate eye coordination and movement.

If a force or blow happens to strike the protruding back center part of the head, the impact may be absorbed by one or both of the occipital lobes. An injury to the crown area (the top of the head) can affect the parietal lobe, which governs spatial awareness and such higher-level visual skills as reading. In either case, bruising, bleeding, swelling, or nerve damage from an MTBI can create havoc within your visual system.

It is important to pin down the source of any vision problems that occur after MTBI. Identifying the culprit helps you to understand your symptoms, know what to expect in terms of recovery, and make decisions about the best course of treatment.

WHAT MTBI-RELATED VISION PROBLEMS ARE LIKE

"I had trouble with double vision after my MTBI, but this problem was eventually found to be a side effect of medication. Over time, I have also experienced blurred, weaker vision in my right eye—the side that was injured. Since

this difficulty seems to be worsened by stress and fatigue, I do what I can to avoid these conditions. Of course, these fluctuations make prescribing and wearing corrective lenses a real problem. On occasion, I'm affected by unexpected light sensitivity, particularly from fluorescent lighting, though it has never been determined whether this problem is related to an injury in my eye or to brain injury. Once in a while, I'm also bothered by floaters."

—D.R.S.

Doctors who work with MTBI patients treat a number of different visual problems, one or more of which may match your own postinjury symptoms. The characteristics of the most common eyesight-related complaints are described in this section.

Blurred Vision

Blurred vision—seeing objects out of focus—after an MTBI can result from damage to the cornea, the transparent membrane covering the front of the eyeball; to the lens, which focuses light on the retina that processes the light image; or to the optic nerve, which transmits visual messages to the brain.

Even if only one eye has been damaged, everything you see will appear blurry. Some cases of blurred vision improve on their own and some can be improved with treatment, but if the blurriness is a result of retinal or optic-nerve damage, you may be left with some permanent degree of blurred vision.

Cortical Blindness

Occasionally, an MTBI involves such severe trauma to both occipital lobes that an intense blurring condition called cortical blindness can result. At worst, this malady allows you to see nothing at all; at best, you may be able to decipher a newspaper headline. Some people eventually regain most of their original sight capacity, though a year or two often passes before it can be determined how much of your sight will return.

Double Vision

Under normal conditions, your eye movements are synchronized so that you see the images reflected on both retinas as a single picture. If the movements of your eyes are affected by nerve damage, however, you may see each retinal image separately—that is, you may see two distinct images instead of one. This phenomenon is called *diplopia*, or double vision.

Double vision makes resuming everyday activities quite difficult and can contribute to headaches, fatigue, and dizziness problems. Double vision may disappear on its own within a period of six weeks or so. However, the condition may linger for a year or longer, or even be permanent, depending on the severity of nerve damage.

Floaters

Floaters—sometimes called *vitreous floaters*—cause moving spots to appear in your field of vision. Occasionally, tiny bits of chemicals or solid matter develop in the vitreous fluid, the clear, protective gel-like substance that fills most of the space in the back half of the eyeball, between the lens and the retina. As these objects move, they reflect light onto the retina. You perceive these reflections as floating spots before your eyes.

Floaters are very common and can occur under ordinary circumstances. Usually, they cause no harm and do not signify a serious problem. When they occur after MTBI, it is often because the injurious blow causes minute hemorrhages within the eye, which result in the formation of numerous small, free-floating solid objects within the gel.

Optic Atrophy

If there is significant trauma to the optic nerve during an MTBI, the nerve is unlikely to heal. It may then begin to atrophy, or waste away. Once this happens, the optic nerve can no longer transmit impulses from the retina to the brain, resulting in blurred vision and significant if not complete vision loss in the affected eye. This permanent loss of vision in one eye in turn hampers your perception of depth and distance.

Photophobia

Sometimes an injury to the visual system results in an unusual sensitivity to light. This condition can manifest itself as anything from seeing an annoying intermittent glare to a crippling intolerance for any sort of light—even through closed eyelids. Light sensitivity can be short-lived or chronic, depending upon the type and severity of injury.

Tracking Problems

Tracking is the ability to follow and maintain your focus on a moving object with both eyes. Tracking problems may result from an injury to the brain stem or the cerebellum. An MTBI in the area of the brain stem sometimes causes *nystagmus,* or rapid oscillations of the eyeball that interfere with smooth, coordinated eye movement when looking to the right, left, up, or down. Slowed eye movement due to MTBI can also cause tracking problems, and can hamper your ability to read or process visual images.

Visual Agnosia

In rare cases, a person who has suffered an MTBI will see an image but be completely unable to attach meaning to it. For instance, you might be handed an apple, but it would remain a meaningless object until you put your senses of touch, smell, and taste to work to help you identify it. This phenomenon, called visual agnosia, can occur during recovery from cortical blindness due to injury to specific areas within the occipital lobes. In its various forms, it can cause spatial confusion; an inability to read, write, draw, or follow a map; or an inability to recognize familiar faces.

Visual Overstimulation

People with MTBI often find themselves visually overstimulated in the months after injury—they cannot tolerate changing light patterns and/or the sight of movement, clutter, or detail. This condition is tied to trauma to one or more areas of the brain responsible for processing images. It may range from intermittent to long-term, from mildly inconvenient to completely incapacitating.

Visual-Field Changes

The visual field is the full extent of your sight capacity when your eyes are looking straight ahead, including your central and side, or peripheral, vision. Sometimes MTBI causes a loss of vision in one area of your visual field. For example, you may clearly see the center of what you are focusing on, but have a blurred or completely missing area to the left or right, depending on the area of the brain that was injured. In some cases, side vision can disappear completely. Left- or right-sided vision loss is generally caused by injury to the visual pathways behind the eyes; central visual-field problems result from injury to one eye or to both of the occipital lobes; and upper or lower visual-field problems stem from damage to the optic nerve.

DIAGNOSING VISION PROBLEMS

Whether mild or severe, temporary or permanent, visual problems that result from MTBI are sure to interfere with many aspects of daily living. If you experience problems with your eyesight in the weeks after your injury, it is a good idea to obtain a thorough evaluation by an ophthalmologist—a medical doctor who specializes in diagnosing and treating eye disorders. This examination will determine the scope and nature of your condition, rule out the possibility of further visual deterioration, and ascertain whether treatment is possible. Based on your diagnosis, your ophthalmologist can also direct you to additional sources of information and support.

TREATING MTBI-RELATED VISION PROBLEMS

There is often no treatment other than time for vision problems resulting from MTBI. Patience may therefore be your doctor's first prescription. Fortunately, some eyesight difficulties eventually diminish or disappear on their own. This is particularly true of problems that arise from injury to the brain, such as cortical blindness, tracking problems, visual agnosia, and visual-field problems. It may take some time, however. For example, recovery from cortical blindness is slow, with vision gradually improving over a two-year period. Similarly, visual-field problems often fade, but it may take as long as a year or two before there is noticeable improvement. With visual agnosia, it is impossible to predict how long healing may take or even what the chances of recovery are.

Any recovery from damage to the optic nerve usually occurs within six months following the injury. After that time, improvement is unlikely. Your ophthalmologist should tell you at what point you should cease to expect any further improvement in your condition.

Of course, many eye problems do respond well to medical, surgical, and alternative approaches. Arming yourself with information about available treatments can help you understand and participate in the healing or coping process, as the case may be. A number of commonly recommended treatments are described below.

Conventional Approaches

Appropriate treatment, if any, for an MTBI-related vision problem depends on the nature of the problem. If blurred vision results from damage to the cornea, antibiotics such as ofloxacin (Ocuflox) and/or anti-inflammatory medications such as prednisone (PredForte) can promote healing. If not, a corneal transplant may be needed to restore your sight.

Prescription eyeglasses are helpful for lens problems, but severe damage may require cataract surgery. An eye patch is often used to help eliminate troublesome double images. If double vision persists for a year or more, surgery on the eye muscles may be done to reposition the eye. Nystagmus is difficult to treat, and time may be the best healer.

In addition to prescribing specific treatments, an opththalmologist can advise you on ways to compensate for visual deficits. If you experience blurriness in your left visual field, for instance, the doctor may suggest that you hold printed matter to the right of your nose when reading to avoid experiencing a blind spot (an area that does not register visual information), or that you turn your head to move your stronger right vision into your left-side blind spot. If you are light-sensitive or suffering from visual overstimulation, your doctor will likely discuss with you ways to avoid painful and distressing visual stimuli. There are no corrective measures for floaters, but most people with floaters eventually become used to them, especially once they settle below the line of sight.

Alternative Approaches

Acupuncture by a qualified licensed acupuncturist may be effective against visual problems such as nystagmus, photophobia, and blurred vision. Various visual problems have been helped by herbal preparations such as bai shao, bilberry, and eyebright. Homeopathics such as *Bryonia album, Gelsemium,* and *Causticum* are also commonly prescribed. As always, what is best for you depends on your specific needs and symptoms. If you are considering such remedies, it is important to consult an herbalist or homeopathic practitioner who can help you, rather than self-prescribing or experimenting with over-the-counter products. If your primary-care physician is unable to help you, or to supply a referral to a qualified herbalist or homeopath, the Herb Research Foundation and/or the National Center for Homeopathy (see the Resources section beginning on page 281) may be able to help.

PRACTICAL SUGGESTIONS

While you wait out the weeks or months necessary to determine the extent of your recovery from MTBI-related vision problems, it pays to do what you can to make yourself comfortable, safe, and better able to cope with day-to-day life. You may find some of the following techniques quite helpful:

- If you have problems with depth perception, use extreme caution when going up or down stairs and curbs. If a handrail is available, use it. Also be cautious when crossing streets—it may be dif-

ficult to tell exactly how much space there is between you and oncoming traffic, or how fast that traffic is approaching.

- Before getting behind the wheel again, have your driving skills assessed to make sure it is safe for you to do so. Tests of this type
are available through most rehabilitation hospitals.

- If reading is a problem, find large-print books and newspapers (or
use a magnifier), and use a ruler to help you keep your place when
reading a printed page. Or make use of audio recordings of books,
magazines, and newspapers from your local public library or Books
on Tape (see the Resources section at the end of the book).

- For computer work, experiment with computer software that reads
aloud to you. Soundproof by HumanWare Inc. may be helpful. This
PC device provides a small voice synthesizer and a tracking system that lets you hear what appears on the monitor rather than
having to read it. Text Assist, a text reader by Creative Labs, Inc.,
is found on most Soundblaster sound cards. (See the Resources section at the back of this book for further information.)

- If you find you have developed light sensitivity, cater to it. Use
dark glasses, keep blinds or shades lowered, and avoid brightly lit
places.

- Avoid becoming visually overstimulated. Choose calm surroundings
over chaotic places such as shopping malls and crowded parties.
Try to sleep during car trips.

- Seek the support of friends and family. Help them understand the
exact nature of your visual problems, delegate responsibilities that
cause you great difficulty, and ask their assistance with environmental and scheduling modifications.

- If you find yourself in a fragile emotional state due to worry and
frustration over eyesight problems, ask your ophthalmologist or primary-care physician about a referral for mental-health assistance.

If your vision remains impaired over the long term as a result of
your MTBI, you may qualify for special services such as job retraining, visual aids, a guide dog, and/or assistance with reorganizing
your home and work space. In most states, your ophthalmologist can
register you for consideration for these benefits. Fortunately, though,
in many cases vision slowly but surely improves after MTBI. Time,
patience, medical advice, and concessions made with your specific visual problem in mind combine to make the recovery period much
easier.

9

HEARING PROBLEMS

John, a 35-year-old sheet-metal worker from South Dakota, was on the job when a tool fell a distance of some six feet and struck him on the top of the head. He immediately began hearing a ringing sound in both ears. John's family physician found no marked hearing loss or visible middle-ear damage. He identified the ringing sound as a neurological consequence of being hit on the head, and said that it would improve in time. Over a year later, however, John was still grappling with the constant sound, most noticeably at night. A neurologist suggested biofeedback, which provided a measure of relief, but John now realizes that he may well have to learn to live with the ever-present ringing in his ears.

Most people tend to associate hearing problems with old age or with damage from middle-ear infections in childhood. As many people with MTBI can attest, however, a force or blow to certain areas of the head also can cause changes in one's ability to hear.

WHY HEARING PROBLEMS CAN OCCUR AFTER MTBI

In a healthy, normal ear, sound waves cause vibrations of the eardrum, which are then transmitted to the the middle ear, and, in turn, to a fluid-filled structure called the *cochlea*, located in the inner ear. In the cochlea, vibrations are changed into electrical impulses that are transmitted to the brain by the auditory, or acoustic, nerves (although certain vibrations, such as those caused by one's own speech, are conducted to the inner ear directly through the skull). The brain interprets these electrical impulses as sound.

Most hearing problems are the result of either conductive failure—

a mechanical problem in the middle ear that keeps vibrations from reaching the cochlea—or sensorineural failure—damage to the inner ear that prevents sound impulses from being relayed to the brain. Typically, these conditions occur as a result of middle-ear fluid entrapment, wax buildup, exposure to noise, and age-related nerve degeneration. However, it is not unusual for a number of hearing problems to arise suddenly after an MTBI.

In some instances, brain trauma is centered in areas of the parietal or temporal lobes that are linked to ear-related functions like balance and spatial awareness or the interpretation of sounds. Usually, however, post-MTBI hearing problems are the result of damage to the middle or inner ear. For instance, an eardrum may rupture. Or there may be swelling around the eustachian tube (a drainage tube that connects the ear to the throat) or bleeding into the middle ear, either of which can cause sound-blocking fluid buildup behind the eardrum. Or tiny, sensitive bones in the middle ear may be destroyed, which also hampers sound transmission. If the cochlea or the surrounding nerves bear the force of impact, all hearing in the affected ear may be lost, or you may become unable to interpret auditory messages.

It is important and reassuring to realize that many MTBI-related hearing difficulties are temporary and treatable. Learning as much as you can about your particular problem can help you take the right steps toward recovery.

WHAT MTBI-RELATED HEARING PROBLEMS ARE LIKE

Trauma to the head or neck can result in a variety of difficulties that either reduce or interfere with your ability to hear, process, or tolerate sounds from your environment. The problems most commonly encountered after MTBI are described below.

Hearing Loss

Hearing loss, or hearing impairment, is a reduction in the ability to hear certain sounds due to nerve damage or a malfunction in the conduction of sound waves in the ear. Low-volume and high-pitched tones are the hardest sounds to hear; rapid or monotone dialogue also is difficult to understand. Hearing loss can rule out comfortable use of the telephone and make everyday interactions quite stressful. In conversation and circumstances in which there is competing noise, you may find yourself having to watch the speaker for clues as to what is being said.

Hearing loss may be temporary or permanent, depending on the cause of the impairment. Fortunately, most types are treatable.

Ménière's Syndrome

This condition, which can occur with or without MTBI, is characterized by one-sided low-frequency hearing loss with a sensation of fullness in the same ear, ringing or buzzing noises in the ear, and severe, even violent, attacks of vertigo (for a detailed discussion of vertigo, see Chapter 6). The amount of hearing loss may fluctuate, and the attacks of vertigo may vary in frequency. When the condition is in full swing, it can effectively render you immobile. While it is known that Ménière's syndrome stems from fluid buildup in the inner ear, there is a great deal of debate as to the underlying cause of this condition. Some treatments that may be suggested include diuretics (medication that alleviates fluid retention), limitation of movement, and, sometimes, surgery to release fluid from the middle ear. At present Ménière's syndrome is incurable, but various symptoms such as vertigo and ringing in the ear are treatable.

Noise Sensitivity

In many cases of inner-ear injury, the body attempts to compensate for loss of function. This can result in extreme sensitivity to loud sounds or noises of a certain pitch. In other cases, MTBI leads to sound-selection problems that render a person unable to discriminate between certain sounds or filter out background noise. Either condition poses a challenge to such everyday activities as conversing in a moving car or following the dialogue in a television program. Further compounding the problem is the fact that noise sensitivity often occurs in conjunction with tinnitus (see below) and hearing loss (see page 98).

Sound Agnosia

In rare cases a condition called sound agnosia, or the inability to comprehend everyday sounds, may occur during recovery from MTBI. This malady is the result of injury to the temporal-parietal area of the brain's right hemisphere (see Chapter 1), and it leaves you able to participate in conversation but unable to identify or locate the source of such ordinary sounds as a ringing doorbell or barking dog. In some cases, there is complete loss of hearing in one ear. Naturally, sound agnosia poses a significant handicap to everyday functioning.

Tinnitus

Like John, in the story at the start of the chapter, many people with MTBI are troubled by tinnitus, or the perception of sounds in the ear that are unrelated to any actual external sound. Ringing and buzzing noises are common. Some people hear fluctuating high-pitched tones like those from the uppermost keys on a pipe organ. Still others hear roaring or hissing noises. The problem is often worse at night or in very quiet surroundings. Needless to say, it can be extremely annoying and, consequently, stressful. MTBI-related tinnitus may be temporary or lifelong.

DIAGNOSING HEARING PROBLEMS

If you experience a hearing problem after an MTBI, it is essential that you be evaluated by an otolaryngologist, or ear/nose/throat (ENT) specialist. Your primary-care physician should be able to refer you to a qualified professional, whose evaluation should include your family and medical histories, a review of the circumstances of your injury, an examination of your ears, and an audiogram, or hearing assessment, by an audiologist. The results will enable the otolaryngologist to establish a diagnosis, prescribe corrective treatment, and suggest techniques to provide relief. He or she can also furnish educational materials and information about support organizations that deal with your particular problem. Because long-term hearing problems can affect speech and language—particularly in children—a referral to a speech/language pathologist may also be in order.

TREATING MTBI-RELATED HEARING PROBLEMS

The nature and severity of a hearing problem are usually good predictors of its curability. Happily, many hearing problems are correctable through a number of approaches. Others respond to a lesser extent to various treatments and practices. What follows is a look at the most successful approaches to hearing problems.

Conventional Approaches

Your doctor will no doubt inform you that many types of hearing problems respond to available medical treatments. For instance, if hearing loss results from damage to the eardrum or inner-ear bones, surgical repair may be in order. Antibiotics and decongestants are often effective at reducing middle-ear fluid buildup that interferes with hearing, as occurs in Ménière's syndrome. In some cases, corrective surgical procedures to drain middle-ear fluid may help to decrease pressure on the vestibular system.

Sound agnosia resulting from MTBI usually resolves itself over time. Tinnitus can be difficult to treat because the exact source of the problem is often impossible to pinpoint. In addition, this problem is often accompanied by hearing loss, and corrective measures for that problem can make tinnitus worse. Antidepressant medication may be used to relieve the emotional stress related to this annoying symptom. If you suffer from tinnitus, it is important to have your doctor assess *all* of the medications you are taking, since dozens of drugs—particularly those containing alcohol—are known to aggravate the condition. An adjustment in your prescription medications may bring significant relief. Hearing aids and tinnitus-masking devices can do a great deal to minimize the effects of long-term hearing problems as well. Thermal biofeedback can help you learn to relax and tune out the annoying sound, while EEG biofeedback can help you consciously alter the brain waves that perceive the sound. Hypnosis may be suggested to help you cope with tinnitus or the psychological effects of hearing impairment. In many cases, the brain eventually becomes used to the constant noise of tinnitus, making the condition less annoying over time.

Alternative Approaches

Certain alternative health practices have been shown to effect improvement in hearing problems such as noise sensitivity and vertigo. Acupressure and both traditional and auricular acupuncture can be particularly helpful. The appropriate type and frequency of treatment varies depending on individual needs and symptoms, so it is necessary to consult with a licensed acupuncturist to determine your specific needs. There are no herbs or homeopathics to eliminate specific symptoms such as tinnitus. However, based on your makeup, there may be remedies that can lessen your symptoms. It is best to consult with a qualified herbalist or homeopathic practitioner to see if help is available to you.

PRACTICAL SUGGESTIONS

As is often the case with MTBI-related symptoms, time can play an important role in correcting your hearing problems. While you follow your doctor's recommendations and wait out the recovery process, there are a number of steps you can take to help minimize the effects of hearing problems on your everyday life:

- Avoid nicotine, caffeine, alcohol, and recreational drugs. These substances have been shown to exacerbate tinnitus.

- Limit your use of salt, which can cause fluid retention and increased vertigo.

- Stick to a regular sleep schedule to reduce stress and anxiety, both of which are tinnitus triggers.

- Sleep with a radio playing softly in the background, or run an electric fan or other source of "white noise" to minimize the effects of tinnitus. There are even alarm-clock-sized noise-generating machines available that are designed specifically for this purpose.

- Call your telephone company's customer service number to inquire about special audio equipment that can make conversing by telephone easier.

- Ask your doctor about the advisability of a lip-reading course. Most rehabilitation facilities offer this type of training.

- Don't hesitate to inform people about sound-selection problems. Ask them to speak one at a time, or find a quiet place to hold conversations.

- Cater to your sound sensitivity by avoiding large-group functions and noisy places. If possible, do your shopping and other necessary errands when public places are least crowded—say, between 10:00 A.M. and noon. If that is not possible, ask a family member to do these chores for you while you are recovering.

- If you find yourself extremely anxious about your hearing problem, ask your doctor about sources of support and psychological help.

The effects of hearing problems on daily living are significant and undeniable. However, it is reassuring to know that many such disorders are cured by time, and that others can be brought under control, if not completely corrected. If your MTBI has left you with hearing difficulties, you can contribute a great deal to your recovery by seeking the expertise of a specialist, taking good physical care of yourself, being forthright about your impairment, and establishing home and work environments in which you can function most comfortably.

10

SENSORY AND METABOLIC DISTURBANCES

Since experiencing an MTBI, Gail, whose story opens Chapter 4, has experienced a variety of sensory and other problems that were not immediately attributed to her injury. For example, certain foods now taste different to Gail, and some cause actual discomfort when eaten. In addition, because she is extremely sensitive to touch, an ordinary act such as opening a jar causes Gail to overreact and jerk her hand back. Cooking—which Gail refers to as a sensory-intensive operation—causes her quite a problem. Surrounded by sights, sounds, and smells, she has to think carefully about every step of the process in order not to feel a sense of overload.

No matter what the activity at hand, Gail is fatigued by too much sensory stimulation, which in her case triggers episodes of double vision and a constant sensation of being cold. She also complains of having a metallic taste in her mouth, and she has gained twenty pounds since her accident. Her doctor attributes the last two problems to her medication.

Have you been annoyed by weight gain or appetite, skin, or sensory problems since your injury? Complaints of this type are common among people with MTBI. By themselves, these miscellaneous symptoms may not seem severe or constant enough to send sufferers to a doctor. And when medical attention *is* sought, sensory and metabolic difficulties are generally viewed as separate from MTBI symptoms. As a result, problems of this nature often go undiagnosed.

The fact is that sensory and metabolic symptoms do occur, either as a direct result of injury to the brain or nearby areas or as a side effect of medication prescribed for other MTBI symptoms.

WHY SENSORY AND METABOLIC PROBLEMS
CAN OCCUR AFTER MTBI

Doctors and researchers do not fully understand the connection between traumatic brain injury and sensory and metabolic difficulties.
However, it is known that even tiny contusions (bruising) in the sensory areas of the brain, which are localized in the parietal, occipital,
and temporal lobes (see Chapter 1), can trigger complaints of this nature. Your MTBI may have damaged nerves that facilitate the sense
of taste or smell, or affected your pituitary gland's hormonal control
of weight and appetite. Injury to the spinal column or nerve receptors in the skin can alter your sense of touch.

SENSORY AND METABOLIC PROBLEMS
THAT CAN FOLLOW MTBI

Sensory and metabolic symptoms vary in type and degree, depending on the nature of your MTBI. Some of the most commonly reported problem areas are described below.

Altered Sense of Smell

*"I was walking to my mailbox one day when I slipped on some ice. I fell
backward without catching myself and hit the right rear of my head on the
cement driveway. My next memory is of twelve hours later, when I found
myself in a Sioux City hospital. When I was served breakfast and lunch the
following day, I blamed the food's tastelessness on institutional cooking. I was
discharged from the hospital with a diagnosis of mild traumatic brain injury
and the recommendation that I see a neurologist within two weeks.*

*At the two-week appointment, my neurologist realized that I had lost my
sense of smell along with most of my sense of taste. He told me not to worry,
for this was a common problem, and my sense of smell would probably return within six weeks. Two weeks after that, I developed a nauseating phantom smell that was very worrisome. Car exhaust and hair sprays in particular triggered a sensation of a strong, unpleasant odor.*

*In the ensuing years, my ability to smell and taste has slowly improved.
However, the phantom odor still intrudes off and on, making my life frustrating and difficult. As it happens, cooking had always been a major part of
my life—in fact, before my injury, I had twice been a finalist in the Pills-
bury Bakeoff. I have had to learn many new coping skills in order to continue entering cooking contests and catering luncheons. Fortunately, my efforts still receive positive reviews."*

—Darlene

Your ability to smell allows you to detect and identify odors. A mild traumatic brain injury can result in *hyposmia* (a partial loss of the capacity to smell) or in *anosmia* (a complete loss of the sense of smell). Another complaint, *dysosmia*, is a change or changes in the sense of smell that cause you to perceive a phantom smell that can be either pleasant, neutral, or, more commonly, distinctly unpleasant. However slight they may be, changes in your ability to smell can be difficult to adjust to.

The sense of smell is probably the least appreciated of all senses. It affects our lives in many ways, not the least of which is our ability to appreciate the flavor of food. Your sense of smell also acts as a signal, alerting you to the presence of such things as gas leaks, spoiled food, and smoke. Dysosmia, or phantom smells, can distract and disgust, while some odors can actually trigger a migraine headache. Research in aromatherapy has shown that our moods, metabolism, and ability to become sexually aroused are all affected by the sense of smell. Clearly, problems in this area can have far-reaching and dramatic effects.

Loss of the Sense of Taste

Under normal circumstances, your tongue can distinguish four basic tastes: sweet, sour, salty, and bitter. However, a disruption along the nerve pathways from the taste buds to the brain can prevent taste messages from being interpreted properly. The result is *hypogeusia*, or decreased ability to taste, while the ability to distinguish food texture, temperature, and spiciness remains intact. Frequently, when a person cannot appreciate the flavor of food, he or she is actually experiencing flavor loss caused by hyposmia or anosmia (see above). Most people with MTBI do retain the ability to detect the irritating properites of certain substances—the burn of chili peppers or the tingle of alcohol, for example.

Changes Involving the Skin

Your skin is your body's largest organ and may undergo changes in sensitivity after an MTBI. Occasional or localized numbness can occur. And, although it is less common, you may experience a heightened sensitivity to touch, sometimes to the point that the feeling of anything—even clothing—touching your skin is unbearable. You may also experience occasional skin rashes or the chronic itching and superficial inflammation of atopic dermatitis, both of which are unexplained but not uncommon results of trauma to the brain.

Appetite and Weight Changes

A decrease in appetite may appear immediately after an MTBI, but this is more common with moderate or severe brain injuries. More characteristic of MTBI is an increase in appetite. Injury to your short-term memory and/or the hypothalamus (the portion of the brain that controls hunger) can play havoc with your appetite, making you feel hungry even when you have just eaten. Also, if you are having problems with short-term memory, you may not *remember* that you have eaten.

An MTBI can also alter your body's metabolism of food, so that you may find that your appetite has increased. Or you may find that you are gaining weight even though your eating habits remain the same because you are now burning calories more slowly. Weight gain can also occur as a side effect of anticonvulsant or other medications, such as antidepressants or sleep aids. Another factor in weight gain is an overall decrease in activity level as a result of chronic fatigue— a major problem after MTBI.

Bladder and Bowel Control Problems

Problems with incontinence (loss of bladder control) and bowel problems such as diarrhea or constipation are embarrassing but not uncommon after MTBI. Brain injury may cause confused messages to be sent to or from the muscles in the bladder and/or the bowel. Incontinence may lead to bladder infections. Constipation may also be caused by inactivity during the period after your MTBI.

DIAGNOSING SENSORY AND METABOLIC PROBLEMS

If your MTBI leaves you with symptoms such as those described above, it is important to tell your neurologist about them. To determine the exact nature of your problem, he or she should do a thorough evaluation, including family and medical histories, a review of the circumstances of your injury, and an examination of the affected area. Additional specialists may be called upon, including an otolaryngologist, a dermatologist, an allergist, or a gastroenterologist.

A comprehensive measure of sensory deficits is best done through an established chemosensory clinic. An institution such as the Taste and Smell Center at the University of Connecticut Health Center (see the Resources section beginning on page 281) can provide a multidisciplinary approach to these problems to determine whether sensory deficits are neurological in origin or not.

Once a diagnosis has been made, your doctor or doctors can prescribe corrective treatment, suggest techniques to provide relief, and furnish educational and support materials.

TREATING MTBI-RELATED SENSORY AND METABOLIC PROBLEMS

"Although I was on a 1,000-calorie, 12-grams-of-fat-a-day diet prescribed by the head of nutrition at a major Boston hospital, I gained over twenty pounds after my MTBI. It was clear that metabolic changes caused by my brain injury, together with side effects of my seizure medication, could override even the healthiest diet. I found going from a well-toned size eight to an out-of-shape size fourteen to be really discouraging, but eventually I decided to focus on the fact that I'm lucky to be alive—although I am still determined to get into the best possible shape for my circumstances by maintaining my healthful eating habits and working out as much as my body will permit."

—D.R.S.

The precise nature and the severity of your symptoms may be good predictors of their curability. Many sensory and metabolic problems reverse themselves over time. Others can be expected to respond to treatment. What follows is a look at the most successful approaches.

Conventional Approaches

Between 5 and 30 percent of people with MTBI lose or face alterations in their sense of smell, sense of taste, or ability to detect common chemicals. However, there are treatments that can help. If the decreased sensory ability is from brain swelling or injury to the nerves for taste or smell, this can be treated with steroids.

If tests indicate that your problem is neurologically based, time will generally be the best healer. There are some medications, such as valproic acid (Depakene), as well as experimental surgical procedures available to treat distorted or phantom smell. Drug treatment for loss of the sense of taste is under research.

In general, skin sensitivity is difficult to treat. EEG biofeedback can sometimes help by changing your perception of sensation. You can also try treating the various symptoms of skin sensitivity with a minor analgesic like acetaminophen (Tylenol, Datril, and others) to reduce pain, an antihistamine such as diphenhydramine (Benadryl) to relieve itching, or aloe vera gel to reduce a dry, uncomfortable feeling.

Treatment for problems with appetite or weight changes caused by MTBI are geared toward the symptoms rather than the cause or injury. Typical approaches may include appetite suppressants and weight-control programs such as Weight Watchers, Jenny Craig, and Diet Workshop. Your neurologist may also recommend consulting a nutritionist who can assist you in revising your diet.

Bodily changes can be very upsetting from an emotional point of view. Cognitive-behavioral therapy can help you cope with weight gain or loss and the sense of having lost control. In some situations, antidepressants may be needed.

Bowel problems can often be helped by increasing water or fluid intake, exercising, and using an over-the-counter stool softener. Incontinence is best treated by a urologist, who may recommend specialized muscle exercises called Kegels (see page 85). There are medications available to help with bladder retraining, but the side effects, such as light sensitivity, can worsen other MTBI symptoms.

Alternative Approaches

Both traditional and auricular acupuncture have been found to be effective against various sensory and metabolic complaints. Acupressure may also be helpful for bladder control. To determine which treatment to use, it is best to consult with a licensed acupuncturist.

There are a number of herbal and homeopathic remedies that may bring some relief. For bladder problems, the herbs sang piao xiao, fu shen, couchgrass, or buchu, or the homeopathic *Nux vomica*, may be helpful. Wu yao is an excellent herb for bowel problems. The homeopathic *Aconitum napellus* or *Natrum muriaticum* may be appropriate for problems with the sense of smell. *Plumbum*, another homeopathic remedy, may be used for skin sensitivity. Before using these or any other alternative remedies, it is best to have a thorough medical evaluation and then to consult with an experienced herbalist or homeopath who has experience in treating people with brain injuries. He or she will be able to prescribe remedies according to your individual needs and symptoms.

PRACTICAL SUGGESTIONS

"When I found myself bothered by skin sensitivity and hot flashes, my doctors first suggested that I stop the medication I was taking at the time. This helped to some extent, but my skin was still more sensitive than usual. My dermatologist suggested experimenting with different detergents and body and facial soaps, and I kept trying different products until I found ones that worked for me."

—D.R.S.

As with many symptoms associated with MTBI, it helps—indeed, it can be necessary—to be inventive and willing to explore alternatives that bring relief. The following suggestions may prove helpful for sensory and metabolic problems:

- Don't assume that your complaint is too minor to mention, or that nothing can be done. Bring sensory and other problems to your doctor's attention.

- Indulge your particular sensitivity. If you are prone to sensory overload, ask for help rather than placing yourself in situations that are physically uncomfortable.

- Experiment with different foods and methods of preparation to determine which tastes or smells are absent or bothersome. Plan meals and snacks around your findings.

- Seek expert help for skin or weight problems. Mainstream corrective measures such as moisturizers or fad diets may not work for you.

- Make sure to have functioning smoke and gas detectors in your home, and keep the batteries current.

- Be exceptionally careful with the preparation of foods and beverages. Refrigerated foods should be date-labeled and stored at appropriate temperatures, and discarded if they look or feel suspicious. When in doubt, have a friend or family member check perishables for spoilage.

- To enhance your enjoyment of food, add texture, contrasting temperatures, and spices. For example, try spicy chips and taco sauce, or ice cream with crunchy nuts and hot syrup.

Bear in mind that you, your MTBI, and your symptoms are completely unique. Listen to your body, and be aware that it may be necessary to experiment in order to find techniques that are effective against sensory and metabolic symptoms. Also keep in mind that even if they are relatively minor, long-term problems of any sort can exact an emotional toll that may impede your recovery. Don't hesitate to ask for medical and family support when you need it.

11

MUSCULAR AND MOTOR PROBLEMS

Bridgeport, Connecticut, residents Helen and Moe, ages 79 and 80, both suffered whiplash when their car was struck in the rear while waiting for a traffic light to change. When the police arrived, Helen complained of facial numbness and severe head pain, and Moe felt neck pain. They were immediately taken to a local hospital for testing. After a brief examination, it was suggested they have physical therapy for their neck spasms. Days later, Helen noticed severe headaches, writing problems, muscle weakness, unsteadiness, and poor coordination in addition to her facial pain and numbness. She was seen by a neurologist, who diagnosed a mild traumatic brain injury and explained that her symptoms were related to her brain injury rather than the whiplash. She was put on Elavil to control her pain.

Nine months later, Moe completed his course of treatment for whiplash, fully recovered. Helen hasn't been as lucky. While physical therapy has eased her neck pain and headaches to some extent, she is still plagued by facial pain and numbness, fatigue, dizziness, continual muscle weakness, poor coordination, unsteadiness, and writing difficulty.

The majority of mild brain injuries result from auto accidents, sports injuries, falls, and physical assaults. In these types of traumas, both the brain and surrounding muscles are affected. The results can interfere with your ability to work, sit, drive, climb stairs, tie your shoes, and do many of the other intricate tasks that most of us do each day without thinking. Muscular injuries from any type of direct trauma are painful and may be slow to heal, but movement problems and chronic central nervous system (CNS) pain from diffuse brain injury may linger even longer or, in some instances, become permanent.

WHY MUSCULAR AND MOTOR PROBLEMS
CAN OCCUR AFTER MTBI

"For over six years, I had chronic neck and shoulder pain from my auto accident. Numerous tests, including nerve conduction, were done to pinpoint the source of my pain. Eventually I was diagnosed with CNS pain that was causing muscle spasm in my neck and shoulder. Various treatments were attempted and proved unsuccessful until I discovered EMG biofeedback. This technique helped stop my muscle spasm and increased my mobility. But it was not until I used EEG biofeedback, which actually changed my pain perception, that my CNS pain stopped completely."

—D.R.S.

The perception of pain is a complex operation that involves an intricate network of connections to and from the spinal cord and brain, which collectively are known as the central nervous system, or CNS. The location of the brain's pain centers and the fine points of pain perception are under research, but it is known that it is the central nervous system that allows you to sense pain when something is not right with your body. In a typical muscle or soft-tissue injury, the brain perceives a warning that the muscle has been injured and sends a message back to the muscle to respond by tightening, or spasming. This in turn causes a pain sensation to be sent back to the brain, completing what is called the pain-spasm cycle.

When there is muscle injury along with brain injury, correctly diagnosing and treating the symptoms becomes extremely complex because the injured brain may still perceive pain long after the muscle injury has healed. This process becomes even more complicated if the body compensates for injury to the motor areas of the brain or to the muscles—or both—by overusing other muscles, which may then also go into spasm.

Diffuse injury to the brain's motor areas, such as the parietal lobe, cerebellum, and brain stem, can directly affect your coordination, strength, balance, muscle tone, and posture. Numbness can be a result of injury to the sensory cortex in the front of the parietal lobe. (For a discussion of the different parts of the brain, see Chapter 1.)

TYPES OF MUSCULAR AND MOTOR PROBLEMS
THAT CAN FOLLOW MTBI

There are several types of muscular and motor problems that can occur as a result of MTBI. Like many effects of brain trauma, these can be intensified by fatigue and other factors. The most frequently cited complaints are described below.

Muscle Coordination

"I had tremendous difficulty with fine motor activities right after my accident. I had a moderate hand tremor and could no longer hold a pen or play my guitar. Several months later, feeling better, I promised my youngest son that I would perform for his class on the last day of school. A long-time guitarist, I never imagined I would have a problem. But to my great embarrassment, my right hand stopped responding in midperformance."

—D.R.S.

Depending on the location and severity of your MTBI, you may have slow, jerky, or uncontrolled movements. You may also encounter tremors—small, involuntary muscular movements that most often affect the head and hands. Even when you know exactly what you want to do—signing your name, threading a needle, or walking up stairs—and you can picture yourself doing it, step by step, in your mind, you may find yourself unable to make your body perform the needed motions. You may also have trouble trying to learn new motor skills, a problem caused by uncoordination or by difficulties with learning or memory (a more detailed discussion of learning and memory problems will be found in Chapter 14).

Muscle Strength

Loss of muscle strength can occur as a result of MTBI if the injured region of the brain is responsible for controlling muscular activity. *Hemiparesis* is the medical term for weakness and difficulty with movement affecting one side of the body. This is most likely to occur with injury that affects one side—the opposite side—of the brain. Paralysis of an entire side, called *hemiplegia*, may occur, although it is uncommon after MTBI. Muscle weakness can also occur due to injury to the muscles themselves or to the nerves that serve them; as a side effect of medications like carbamazepine (Atretol, Tegretol); or as a result of sleep problems.

Perhaps the most common cause of muscle weakness after MTBI is simple disuse atrophy resulting from inactivity. While this problem is not painful, it can disrupt the range of your daily activities.

Muscle Tone

Brain injury can affect muscle tone, which is the tightness of the muscles when they are at rest. When muscle tone is normal, your body moves smoothly and easily. Injury to a CNS motor area can cause muscle tone to be too tight. You may experience muscle spasm, or tightening of a single muscle or muscle group, or hypertonicity, the tensing of all muscles, which causes your limbs and trunk to stiffen. Because muscle spasm is also the bodily response to pain, it can be difficult to determine whether the problem is from a brain injury or a muscle injury.

Posture

Brain injury can affect the muscles that control your head, neck, shoulders, and the rest of your body. If your neck muscles are in spasm from a brain or muscle injury, this can cause your body to go out of proper alignment, resulting in limited range of motion, muscle weakness, pain, and reduced muscle tone.

Both body movements and posture involve your bones, joints, and surrounding soft tissues—specifically, your muscles, tendons, and ligaments. If a joint between two bones is placed in a position that overstretches the surrounding soft tissues, injury occurs. This is true for all joints in your body, but has particular importance where the spine is concerned. In the spine, the soft tissues also support the soft discs that separate and cushion the vertebrae. Therefore, determining whether a posture problem is due to brain injury or direct bodily trauma is extremely difficult.

Muscle Injuries

There are several muscular problems that can occur after MTBI. In these cases, the brain injury does not cause the injury to the muscles; rather, the same head trauma that results in brain injury also causes injuries to the muscles and tendons near the impact area. Understanding the origin and nature of your particular complaint can help you understand your discomfort. The most frequently cited muscle injuries occurring in association with MTBI are discussed below.

Whiplash

The impact of a blow to the head can cause stretching and tearing of the neck muscles, tendons, and ligaments, because of hyperextension (excessive backward motion) or hyperflexion (excessive forward motion) of the cervical (upper) spine. This type of injury is most often a result of a motor vehicle accident or sports collision. Pinched or damaged nerves may occur, along with injury to the neck muscles, tendons, and joint-stabilizing ligaments, resulting in acute or chronic pain. Muscle damage that leads to the formation of adhesions (scars that form unnatural attachments between tissues or structures in the body) between or within the muscles can prohibit free movement of the head and trigger painful spasms affecting the upper back, neck, face, and/or jaw muscles.

Myofascial Dysfunction

This problem is an offshoot of whiplash that involves the muscles surrounding the neck, some of which continue up into the face. With this type of injury, the fascia, a cellophane-like membrane between the muscles, can become scarred to the muscle, resulting in restricted movement of the neck and facial muscles, and pain that radiates into the face, jaw muscles, cheek, arm, and/or hand.

Fibromyalgia

This muscle-pain syndrome—once known as fibrositis, myofascial pain syndrome, or psychogenic rheumatism—often develops following injuries to the neck and back. Localized or radiating pain may be traced to walnut-sized tender nodules, called "trigger points," within certain muscles. This condition often affects muscles of the neck, shoulder, buttocks, or anywhere along the spine. Pressure on a trigger point produces local tenderness as well as pain that radiates upward to the back of the head, or outward into the upper arm or thigh. The exact cause of these symptoms is unknown, but it is known that they can be aggravated by stress.

Temporomandibular (TM) Disorders

This is another type of muscular problem associated with whiplash. TM disorders, formerly called TMJ syndrome, include a variety of painful conditions of the temporomandibular (jaw) joint and muscles. Other complaints sometimes accompany the TM condition, including pain and a sensation of fullness in the ear, tinnitus, dizziness, and even hearing loss. The fact that these symptoms suggest problems within the ear can make it very difficult to identify TM disorders.

DIAGNOSING MUSCULAR AND MOTOR FUNCTION PROBLEMS

Most people who experience MTBI receive little or no professional evaluation of muscular or motor function immediately afterward. Treatment usually focuses on obvious physical injuries, if any—broken bones, cuts and bruises, and the like. If you can walk and talk normally, it is often assumed that all is well.

Later, if you go to your physician complaining of motor and/or muscular difficulties along with chronic pain, your primary-care physician may refer you to an orthopedist, physiatrist, or neurologist for evaluation and rehabilitation. These specialists may prescribe further diagnostic tests, such as a CT scan or MRI (see Chapter 2). If you have complaints involving an ear, you may also need to see an oto-laryngologist (ear, nose, and throat doctor), who will do a structural assessment and hearing test. Other diagnostic tests commonly used to assess muscular and motor difficulties are described below.

Flexion/Extension X-Rays

This diagnostic test involves x-raying the neck or back during flex-ion, or bending forward, and extension, or bending backward. This can identify bone misalignment, such as two or more vertebrae out of normal position due to ligament or muscle damage.

Electromyography and Nerve Conduction Velocity Study

Electromyography (EMG) and the nerve conduction velocity (NCV) study are used to investigate where damage has occurred in nerves supplying the various muscles in the body. The EMG may be com-pared to testing the wiring in a wall of your house to investigate why the light switch is not working; it measures the electrical activ-ity in the muscles to determine whether the nerves that serve the muscles in the injured part of the body are intact and the muscles are functioning normally. A thin insulated needle is inserted into the muscle and measurements of electrical discharges are taken while the muscle is at rest and at work. The EMG is usually done in the hand or foot, though other locations on the body are sometimes used.

The NCV study is similar to checking the speed with which elec-trical current travels from the power plant to the light switch. In this test, the speed and frequency of electrical impulses from your brain or spinal cord to the injured muscles are measured. A nerve is mild-ly shocked at one location and the response is measured at another location. Slower than normal conduction of nerve impulses can indi-cate nerve damage.

Both of these tests are often experienced as being uncomfortable, even painful. The doctors who administer these tests are aware of this, however.

Myelography

In this test, radio-opaque dye is injected into the spinal canal and x-rays are taken that show the dye as a white substance outlining the disc and nerve roots. This is done to pinpoint disc or nerve damage and scar tissue. The myelogram is more effective at finding lesions than either the CT scan or MRI. However, because it is invasive, it is used less often.

Physical Capacity Evaluation

This consists of a series of timed tests to evaluate your balance, muscle tone, muscle strength, coordination, and flexibility. You may be asked to carry a box around a room, balance on a platform, or pick up small items. To measure grip strength, there is a small device that you squeeze with either hand. A physical capacity evaluation is usually done by a physical therapist or at a rehabilitation hospital.

Thermography

This test involves taking an infrared photograph of the surface of the body using a camera with heat-sensitive film. A thermograph detects temperature differences in different parts of the body. These may be caused by injuries to nerves or blood vessels at the site of pain.

Even with modern diagnostic testing, it can sometimes be difficult to differentiate between brain injury that causes specific muscle, tendon, and ligament problems and direct injury to those same areas—particularly if chronic pain is involved. Your doctor will try to distinguish among the different tissue injuries, movement problems, and types of chronic pain, and prescribe appropriate treatment based on his or her assessment.

Fibromyalgia in particular is difficult to pin down, because the disorder leaves no neurological or orthopedic indicators on standard diagnostic tests. Some physicians will diagnose fibromyalgia if they can induce pain by applying pressure at several specific trigger points in various muscles throughout the body. Identifying temporomandibular disorders is another challenge, because the physical and ear examinations that are usually done in response to a patient's complaints typically yield only negative results. Myofascial dysfunction also can be difficult to diagnose because its symptoms can mimic (or coexist with) those of other disorders, including herniated disc, joint syndromes, and displaced vertebrae.

TREATING MTBI-RELATED MUSCLE AND MOTOR PROBLEMS

Depending on your physical makeup and the force of your injury, you may recover within a few weeks without treatment or suffer longer-term complications as a result of brain injury or nerve damage. In either case, recovery may be interrupted by setbacks and is rarely uniform.

Conventional Approaches

Various types of rehabilitative work can help to overcome motor difficulties, as well as chronic pain. Physical therapy techniques help with balance, motor coordination, muscle movement, tone, spasm, and strength. This type of therapy is also helpful in treating general inflammation and myofascial pain. For more extensive rehabilitation, you might need to see a physiatrist, a medical doctor who specializes in physical medicine and rehabilitation.

Specialized treatment such as biofeedback can be obtained through rehabilitation-hospital programs for people with mild brain injury. Biofeedback can be extremely helpful in many situations. Thermal and EMG biofeedback can increase muscle responsiveness and coordination, as well as helping to control discomfort. EEG biofeedback can help to normalize electrical activity in the motor areas of the brain, enhancing motor reflexes and changing the perception of pain. Hypnosis and relaxation training can also be effective for pain management. However, all three of these techniques—biofeedback, hypnosis, and relaxation training—can present a challenge for people with concentration or attention-span difficulties.

There are various types of indirect physical therapy treatment designed to heal and strengthen muscles and improve balance, coordination, and flexibility. One of these, the Burdenko method, involves dynamic water- and land-based movement exercises. The water portion is done in a vertical position using flotation devices to help you achieve natural traction, allowing gravity to gently separate the vertebrae. The land exercises are an extension of these therapeutic movements. To find a qualified Burdenko therapist in your area, refer to the Resources section beginning on page 281.

Another form of indirect physical therapy, the Feldenkrais method, is a series of subtle exercises designed to retrain your body's movement patterns for pain control and more efficient motor function. A practitioner teaches you alternative ways of moving to replace faulty patterns that may aggravate your injury. To find a qualified Feldenkrais therapist in your area, refer to the Resources section beginning on page 281. Therapeutic horseback riding—a relatively new technique—also enhances balance, coordination, and physical stability.

Movement and dance therapy are forms of dynamic therapy that force the brain to adapt to injury by learning to use different parts than previously to facilitate motor movement. This helps the brain to form new nerve connections to replace those impaired by injury. Music and dance therapy incorporate multiple movements and sensory input, and are available through many colleges, special-education services, and dance studios.

If you need to overcome small motor impairments, or learn new techniques for dispatching troublesome tasks at home and at work, occupational therapy may be recommended. As an alternative, you may choose to undergo cognitive retraining, which involves learning new ways of accomplishing tasks that have become problematic. Or you may choose vocational therapy to learn skills that will prepare you to seek a different type of employment.

Chronic pain, whether from brain injury or from muscle spasm, can have a significant impact on your quality of life. Drug therapy is the usual starting place for people who are trying to cope with pain. After an MTBI, however, you should bear in mind that you may be newly sensitive even to low doses of over-the-counter products. In addition, side effects—a fact of life with any medication—can play havoc with your recovery, so be sure to start with minimal doses and follow your doctor's instructions carefully.

Minor aches and pains are best treated with aspirin and/or nonsteroidal anti-inflammatory drugs (NSAIDs) like ibuprofen and naproxen sodium. These products block the production of body chemicals called prostaglandins, which play an important role in the pain, heat, and swelling that occurs with tissue damage. Prescription-strength NSAIDs are available for people who do not respond to over-the-counter drugs.

Prescription medications used by pain sufferers also include diazepam (Valium), which is used as a muscle relaxant, and amitriptyline (Elavil, Endep), an antidepressant also used for pain management. It is still unclear how and why these medications work to reduce pain; however, they have been found to be very effective in some cases. Corticosteroid injections may be used for treatment of joint pain, particularly in the hands, ankles, feet, hips, or knees.

Narcotics, which block the transmission of pain messages to and from the brain and spinal cord, are an option for extremely severe, persistent pain. If you require more powerful pain medication such as the narcotic meperidine (Demerol), you may be able to reduce the amount you need if you supplement the prescription drug with over-the-counter medication such as aspirin, acetaminophen (Tylenol, Datril, and others), ibuprofen (Advil, Motrin, Nuprin, and others), and/or naproxen sodium (Aleve). By alternating among different products, you are more likely to stay on lower doses of medications. Keeping your use of powerful prescription medications to a minimum has several beneficial effects. First, it helps to prevent your body from building up a tolerance to the drug, which would make you require progressively stronger and stronger pain relief. Second, it helps to keep side effects to a minimum. In addition, taking an over-the-counter product in conjunction with a prescribed pain medication—with your doctor's approval, of course—can sometimes enhance the prescription drug's effectiveness. Furthermore, matters can be complicated by rebound phenomenon, in which increasing the dose of pain medication can actually cause additional pain as the medication begins to wear off.

A form of continuous administration, called *epidural therapy,* involves the injection of narcotics directly into the membrane around the spinal cord. This helps to avoid numerous side effects associated with these drugs.

There are several nonmedicinal pain-control options available as well. *Transcutaneous electrical nerve stimulation,* or TENS, involves the wearing of a small battery-powered generator that transmits electrical impulses to underlying nerves. This electrical activity can block pain signals traveling to the brain, and may also stimulate your body's production of natural pain-control substances. Cognitive-behavioral therapy can help you ward off depression, manage stress, and find the emotional tools for coping with long-term pain. However, both hypnosis and relaxation training can present a challenge for people with concentration or attention-span difficulties.

Alternative Approaches

Chiropractic adjustments can help to realign vertebrae in the neck, thus improving blood flow and nerve-impulse supply to problem muscles. This approach also allows for freer movement and more space between the joints. Polarity therapy, which maximizes the flow of internal energy and encourages the body to heal itself, may be effective against muscle and movement problems. Some people believe that reorganizing the body's energy structure, internal flow, and communication mechanisms can help improve balance and coordination. Acupuncture has been found to be very effective with chronic pain and muscle spasm.

Both herbal and homeopathic preparations are available for pain relief. Herbal remedies sometimes recommended for pain include white willow bark, bai shao, and ye jaio. Among homeopathics, *Arnica* can relieve muscle soreness, while *Natrum sulphuricum, Bungaris,* and *Carbo vegetabilis* help with balance, muscle tone, and strength. Before trying any over-the-counter herbal or homeopathic remedy, it is best to consult with an herbalist or homeopathic practitioner who knows your specific problems and needs.

PRACTICAL SUGGESTIONS

"Three years after my accident, I was still struggling with stability, balance, and walking. While in Switzerland, I discovered a telescoping walking stick that collapses to twelve inches in length and extends to almost four feet, and has straps and hand grips. In light of my balance problem, the Swiss shopkeeper advised me to use two sticks. Walking in the woods with only my hiking sticks has given me a wonderful feeling of freedom!"

—*D.R.S.*

"What works for me is a pen with a fat barrel, such as the Shaefer Big Red, and a Mead fiber-tipped pen."

—*Barbara*

"I still have difficulty remembering motor movements in my rehab program. I've found that when I feel a movement and sense it through a rhythmic beat, I can perform it immediately and remember it even days later."

—*D.R.S.*

Muscular and motor difficulties can wreak havoc with almost every activity on your daily agenda. While the prognosis for recovery is often quite good, the healing process can take time. In the meantime, there are steps you can take to make your life easier and more comfortable:

- If self-care tasks prove difficult during the early phase of your recovery, consider hiring a home health aide.

- Shop with an eye toward making home and personal care tasks easier. Look for items with Velcro closures or large handles, for instance. The Resources section, beginning on page 281, lists catalogues that can help you find a wide array of items designed specifically for people with muscular and motor problems. A rehabilitation hospital can also help you.

- If fine motor problems make writing difficult, trying using a clipboard and felt-tipped or wide-barreled pen to make this task easier. Also consider using a slip-on pencil grip and number-three pencils, which have harder lead than customary pencils. If writing by hand is temporarily out of the question, use a computer or word processor instead.

- Join a local support group or communicate by computer with people affected by symptoms similar to yours. Through such contacts you can gain valuable advice, as well as emotional and psychological support, from others who have "been there." The wisdom and encouragement of others in your situation can be extremely helpful.

- Remember that a cycle of muscle deconditioning and weakness begins after only a few days of bed rest. Avoid what may become months of reconditioning therapy by engaging in whatever light activity you can manage.

- Avoid tension and stress, which place more strain on joints and muscles and may cause additional discomfort.

- Try hot or cold packs to help numb or loosen muscles in the affected area. Warm baths or showers can also be very effective.

The pain that follows an MTBI can indeed be difficult to live with. However, a positive attitude is one of the keys to a faster recovery. Chances are good that the weeks and months after injury will be much easier to bear if you refuse to be victimized by pain. Instead, retake control of your life by working with your health-care provider and searching for your own creative solutions to chronic discomfort.

12

SEIZURES

Beverley was on her way home from a gymnastics meet when she lost control of her car. The car fishtailed, accelerated, flew over a snowbank, and landed sideways. Beverley suffered a mild traumatic brain injury and spent two weeks in an acute-care hospital before being sent to a rehabilitation hospital for ten weeks. She was discharged from there with the assurance that her various problems would go away with time.

Twelve months later, while volunteering at the rehabilitation hospital, Beverley had a seizure. Within twenty-four hours, she had two more. Her diagnosis at the time was either a stroke in the left brain or a seizure with paralysis. Her neurologist put her on Tegretol, an anticonvulsant (anti-seizure) medication. Unlike many people who have seizures, Beverley experiences no auras, peculiar smells, or other signs warning of an oncoming seizure. As a result, her medication level must be kept high so that she can continue to drive. Unfortunately, the medication severely limits both her creative expression and sex drive.

There is neither rhyme nor reason to Beverley's seizures. Sometimes she loses the thread of conversation at one point and picks it up at another. Other times, she has no lapse of memory but simply falls to the floor. Usually she has no recollection of what happens during her seizures and is confused and disoriented when she comes to. Beverley suspects that she experienced seizure activity in the weeks before her second hospitalization but never knew what was happening. Only when her seizures occurred in the presence of a professional trained in treating brain injury was the problem identified and treated. For that, Beverley considers herself lucky.

Seizures are not as rare as you might think. Sometimes called *ictal events,* they involve a sudden, temporary, unusual discharge of electrical impulses in one focal area of the brain that may quickly spread, or diffuse, causing uncontrolled stimulation of nerves and muscles. Seizures can result in abnormal or arrested movement, alteration of consciousness, disorders of sensation or perception, and behavior disturbances. People can develop seizures due to birth defects, metabolic or circulatory disorders, brain tumors, or brain injury. Often, the cause of seizures is unknown. Recurrent seizures are termed *epilepsy*, a condition that affects one percent of the general population. Epilepsy that results from injury is called *posttraumatic epilepsy*. Brain injury is the leading cause of posttraumatic epilepsy in teenagers and young adults.

In general, seizures do not cause brain damage unless they last longer than thirty minutes—a circumstance that is extremely rare with MTBI. However, inherent in seizure disorder is a loss of control that is particularly dismaying to people with MTBI, many of whom are already wrestling with other aftereffects of brain trauma that may make them feel they have lost control of their lives.

WHY SEIZURES CAN OCCUR AFTER MTBI

Seizures, one of the most serious consequences of brain trauma, are most often associated with moderate and severe brain injury. However, they do sometimes occur after a mild traumatic brain injury as well. Neurologists are not entirely sure what causes the irregular discharge of energy that produces seizures in such cases, but some speculate that trauma excites nerves within the brain, causing them to go out of rhythm. Seizures, then, are the body's efforts to correct this irregularity. Another theory is that the misfiring of electrical signals after MTBI stems from bleeding or shearing of nerves within the brain.

In some cases, this unusual discharge of energy takes place across almost all of the brain, causing a *generalized seizure* to take place. Other times, irregular impulses are limited to one section of the brain, resulting in what is termed a *partial seizure*. There are also *unilateral seizures*, which affect only one side of the brain (and, therefore, the body), and *unclassified seizures*, for which no specific location can be pinpointed. In most instances, a given individual will have only one type of seizure problem.

Seizures often originate in the temporal lobes (see Chapter 1). This part of the brain is particularly vulnerable to seizure-causing damage because the structures within it require high levels of oxygen, the blood supply to the area is easily disrupted, and it is located very close to the hard skull. In fact, complex partial seizures so often originate in this area of the brain that you may hear them referred to as *temporal-lobe seizures*. Less frequently, seizure activity may also involve the frontal, occipital, or parietal lobes.

If you experience seizures as a result of MTBI, there are often contributing circumstances. For example, a family history of seizures may give you a propensity for this type of irregular electrical activity, enabling even a mild jolt to your brain to act as a trigger. Or you may have suffered meningitis or seizures in childhood, or had a previous brain injury. Overuse of drugs or alcohol can also be a factor in the development of seizures. Research shows that the risk of seizures continues for at least ten years after an MTBI, and increases significantly if a seizure occurs shortly after the injury.

Certain physical, external, and internal events can act as seizure triggers—that is, they can cause irregular impulses to begin. Physical triggers can include medications, alcohol, and illness, as well as certain light or sound patterns. There are also external triggers that stem from situations in the home, work, or school environment, and internal triggers that can ignite the same chain of events from within. A list of common seizure triggers appears in Table 12.1.

WHAT MTBI-RELATED SEIZURES ARE LIKE

The symptoms that accompany MTBI-related seizures differ from person to person, depending on the pattern and spread of the irregular electrical discharge in the brain. Technically, there are four classes of seizures—generalized, partial, unilateral, and unclassified—as outlined above, plus a number of subdivisions within each category. However, medical experts often characterize seizures as either generalized or partial. The kinds of seizures most often associated with MTBI are absence seizures, tonic-clonic seizures, and simple and complex partial seizures. Other types of seizures, not commonly associated with MTBI, include akinetic, atonic, and myoclonic seizures.

Absence Seizures

These are generalized seizure events that were once termed *petit mal* (literally, "little illness") to distinguish them from seizures that result in full-body convulsions. Absence seizures do not cause muscular spasms or twitching, but instead cause a brief disruption of consciousness. You may suddenly stop speaking or stare blankly for a moment, and then resume the activity at hand—often without being aware of the break in attention.

Tonic-Clonic Seizures

Tonic-clonic seizures are generalized seizures, once referred to as *grand mal* ("great illness") seizures, that cause you to lose consciousness and shake and twitch uncontrollably. Your muscles convulse for several min-

Table 12.1 Common Seizure Triggers

Type of Trigger	Examples
Physical	Holding your breath
	Hyperventilating
	Illness, fever, injury, or pain
	Insufficient sleep
	Missed medications
	Menstruation
	Over- or underexertion
	Overuse of alcohol or stimulants
	Poor nutrition or skipped meals
	Specific light, sound, or touch patterns (flashing lights, for example)
	Withdrawal from alcohol or drugs
External	Arguments
	Criticism
	Death of a loved one
	Failure
	Overwork
	School, job, marital, or financial pressures
	Threatened loss of relationship
	Threatened loss of job
Internal	Agitation
	Anger
	Anxiety
	Boredom
	Depression
	Excitement
	Fear
	Feelings of inadequacy
	Grief
	Tension
	Worry

utes, after which movement subsides and you awaken with no memory of the incident. You are likely to feel dazed, confused, and sleepy, but in most cases can resume your previous activities after resting.

Simple Partial Seizures

Sometimes described as *focal seizures,* these take place without impairment of consciousness. Partial seizures can involve autonomic symptoms, such as fluctuations in your heart rate or blood pressure;

sensory symptoms, such as hearing or seeing things that are not present; or motor symptoms—most often a sudden, jerky movement of one part of your body.

Complex Partial Seizures

Complex partial seizures take place when an extra discharge of electrical energy in the brain propels electrical impulses to certain parts of the brain but without involving the entire organ. A complex partial seizure may cause symptoms such as numbness or muscle weakness. You usually experience an alteration of consciousness, sometimes associated with motor or sensory symptoms. Your level of awareness decreases, but you do not lose consciousness. Additional symptoms can include sensations such as butterflies in the stomach, changes in heart rhythm, and tingling in the face or arms.

Auras

Regardless of the type of seizures you have, you may experience a phenomenon known as an *aura* shortly before the onset of the seizure itself. This is an unusual feeling that acts as a warning that an electrical discharge is about to take place in the brain. Auras may be experienced in many different ways—as changed thinking, reasoning, perception, sensation, or body movement. You may have a feeling of *déjà vu*, a recurrent daydream, or a rush of paranoia. Occasionally, involuntary muscle movement is also involved. The type of aura you experience depends on the area of the brain from which the seizure originates (see Figure 12.1).

Interictal Behavior Syndrome

After a seizure, you are likely to feel disoriented and fatigued. This is called *postictal* (or sometimes *interictal*) behavior. You may feel spacy and confused, but this is usually temporary and disappears after a period of rest.

Interictal behavior syndrome (IBS), on the other hand, denotes a longer-term, more dramatic personality difference exhibited by some seizure sufferers. The syndrome is often characterized by biological changes, such as depression, diminished sexuality, or increased aggression. An affected individual may also become preoccupied with mystical thinking or feelings of extrasensory perception, or become unusually wordy and obsessed with details. In addition, IBS can trigger emotional changes such as social clinginess, the need to express oneself in writing, or difficulty ending conversations. It is believed

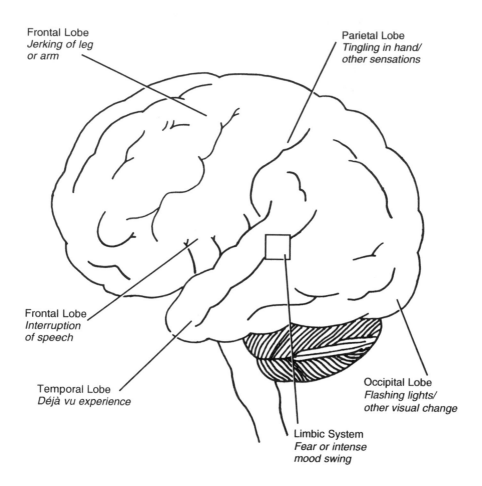

Figure 12.1 Types of Auras and Their Origins in the Brain

gression. An affected individual may also become preoccupied with mystical thinking or feelings of extrasensory perception, or become unusually wordy and obsessed with details. In addition, IBS can trigger emotional changes such as social clinginess, the need to express oneself in writing, or difficulty ending conversations. It is believed that IBS results from progressive changes in the brain stem caused by recurrent seizure activity. Research suggests that irregular discharges may have a kindling effect—that is, a discharge in one part of the brain may cause a stirring of electrical impulses in another area.

DIAGNOSING SEIZURES

Since many of the symptoms of migraine headaches mimic those of addition, some of the manifestations of seizure activity can be symptoms of more than one kind of ictal event. While you might expect symptoms to overlap in this way, considering the complex neurological problems involved, this can make it difficult to categorize seizures.

If you suspect that you might be experiencing seizures as a result of your MTBI, it is imperative that you ask your primary-care physician for a referral to a neurologist who specializes in epilepsy. This specialist will ask you for an in-depth medical history and give you a thorough neurological examination. He or she will probably perform an EEG to determine the focal point, nature, and frequency of any irregular electrical impulses within your brain. Your symptoms will also be considered. The neurologist may suggest additional diagnostic testing, such as an MRI or CT scan, to determine whether there is any structural damage to the brain (see Chapter 2 for an explanation of these diagnostic procedures).

TREATING MTBI-RELATED SEIZURES

It is important to realize that while seizures can usually be suppressed, they cannot be cured. However, you can gain a sense of control over this disorder by determining whether certain events or circumstances tend to set off your seizure activity. You may find it helpful to keep a record of your surroundings, activities, experiences, and moods over a number of days. Also make a note of all food, drink, and medications you consume. Then record the approximate times of any suspected seizures. Share all of this data with your specialist.

The approach taken toward seizure management is usually based on whether part or all of your brain is involved. Typical courses of treatment are described below.

Conventional Approaches

"After my accident, I experienced intermittent facial numbness, motor problems, and postictal behavior. Despite the fact that I had never had an abnormal EEG, based on my symptoms my neurologist felt that I was having partial seizures involving the temporal lobe, cerebellum, and reticular formation system. I was placed on Tegretol, an anticonvulsant medication, and had a toxic reaction that caused me to become highly agitated and see four of everything. The dosage was lowered and these symptoms went away, but months later, I began noticing muscle weakness. I was taken off Tegretol and started on Depakote, another anticonvulsant. On this medication, I gained twenty pounds, felt spacy all the time, and had periods of imbalance, slurred speech, and lightheadedness. Eventually, I was gradually weaned from anticonvulsant

medication and showed marked improvement in memory, balance, and endurance."

—D.R.S.

Anticonvulsant medication is the primary treatment for seizures. Of course, your biological makeup and MTBI are unique, and these medications can cause side effects such as sleepiness, stomach upset, anxiety, and fluctuations in heart rate. Therefore, your medication and dosage must be tailored to meet your individual needs. The goal is to inhibit seizures with the fewest possible side effects, and without compounding other MTBI aftereffects. While multiple medications are sometimes necessary, the use of a single medication at the lowest possible dosage is the method of choice. A trial-and-error approach is often necessary to find the right medication and dosage, so it is important that your neurologist be available for consultation about any problems you encounter.

Generalized seizures are often treated with phenytoin (Dilantin) and phenobarbital; partial seizures with beta-blockers, carbamazepine (Atretol, Tegretol), and divalproex sodium (Depakote). (For a more complete list of anticonvulsant medications, see Table 12.2). It is not fully understood how these medications work, but it is known that they somehow inhibit the excessive electrical discharges that are responsible for seizures. The prescribed amount and frequency of medication depend on such factors as your weight, age, other drugs taken regularly, and your sensitivity to drugs in general.

If you must take anticonvulsant medication, you should become familiar with such terms as *drug level* (sometimes also called *serum level*), which refers to the amount of medication in the liquid portion of your blood at any one time. It is also important to understand about a drug's *half-life,* which is the amount of time it takes for half of a dosage of a drug to be metabolized—that is, to become inactivated—within your body. A drug's half-life can vary widely from person to person; therefore, calculating the speed at which your body inactivates a particular drug is critical to determining the appropriate dosage, and is also important when mixing or discontinuing medications. If too much medication accumulates within your body, you may experience signs of toxicity, with symptoms that can include breathing or visual problems, anxiety, tremors, skin rashes, impaired memory, and heart rhythm problems. You may also be allergic to a particular medication and suffer symptoms ranging from skin rash to arthritis to cardiac arrest. In addition, if you must take an anticonvulsant, you should always remember the following points:

• Be aware that over-the-counter medications can interfere with the

Table 12.2 Anticonvulsant Medications

Generic Name (Brand Name)	Type of Seizures Treated
Carbamazepine (Atretol, Tegretol)	Complex partial; simple partial; tonic-clonic
Clonazepam (Klonopin)	Akinetic; myoclonic
Divalproex sodium (Depakote)	Absence; atonic; myoclonic; tonic-clonic
Ethosuximide (Zarontin)	Absence
Mephobarbital (Mebaral)	Complex partial; simple partial; tonic-clonic
Phenobarbital	Complex partial; simple partial; tonic-clonic
Phenytoin (Dilantin)	Complex partial; simple partial; tonic-clonic
Primidone (Mysoline)	Complex partial; simple partial
Valproic acid (Depakene)	Absence; atonic; myoclonic; tonic-clonic

action of anticonvulsant drugs. Consult your doctor before using any nonprescription product.

• Remember that anticonvulsant medications can neither prevent nor reverse interictal behavior syndrome. In some cases, the use of these drugs may increase depression or other emotional conditions.

• Never discontinue a medication on your own. Doing so can sometimes trigger potentially damaging seizures. If you have problems and complaints about your medication, bring them to your doctor's attention.

Besides treating your seizures medically, your doctor can direct you to support professionals. For instance, he or she might recommend a counselor who specializes in coping with epilepsy, or support groups for you and your family. You might also consider consulting a psychiatrist or psychologist who specializes in behavioral medicine (see Chapter 3). Biofeedback has been shown to be very effective at controlling seizures. Progressive relaxation can help you manage emotional triggers.

For varying reasons, a small percentage of seizures do not respond to anticonvulsants. In rare situations in which seizure activity is uncontrollable, surgery may be necessary to remove the focal area. If all else fails, you may wish to consult your doctor about the feasibility of such approaches as megadoses of vitamin B$_6$, various mineral supplements, and special diets. One specialized dietary program called the *ketogenic diet* (so named because it results in the presence of high levels of substances called ketones in the body) is one of the oldest forms of therapy for epilepsy, and has been used with considerable success to control seizures. However, it has largely fallen into disuse because of the availability of anticonvulsants.

Alternative Approaches

Certain herbs, such as black cohosh, hyssop, and lobelia, are commonly included in herbal prescriptions for people who suffer from seizures. *Circuta virosa, Helleborus,* and *Natrum sulphuricum* are homeopathic remedies that may be prescribed for seizures that are related to brain injury. However, taking self-prescribed over-the-counter herbs or other remedies may not always produce the desired result, leading to the mistaken conclusion that herbal or homeopathic treatments are not useful. Worse, some herbal preparations may actually contribute to seizures in susceptible people. MTBI and seizure disorders are complex problems. It is therefore crucial to consult with, and use such alternative remedies under the guidance of, a well-trained herbalist or homeopathic practitioner who understands and has worked with seizure disorders and MTBI (*see* Assessing a Practitioner's Expertise With MTBI, page 45).

PRACTICAL SUGGESTIONS

Living with an MTBI and its symptoms is no small task. This challenge is greatly compounded if the aftereffects you suffer include seizures. However, there are things you can do to improve your sense of control over this problem—enough so that you can lead a fairly normal life. The following suggestions may help:

- Take all prescribed medications exactly as directed. If you feel a particular medication is causing you problems, consult your physician. *Do not* discontinue a drug or increase or decrease the dosage on your own.

- If you drive, consult your doctor about the advisability of continuing to do so.

- Avoid sports and activities that could be dangerous to yourself or others until your seizure medication and dosage have been regulated.

- Avoid all alcohol. Also avoid caffeine, nicotine, and other stimulants.

- Avoid missed sleep and unnecessary stress—both conditions that can trigger seizures.

- Be honest about your seizures. Dealing with your condition in a forthright manner helps to make others more comfortable and can generate valuable support.

Recovery from posttraumatic epilepsy due to MTBI is variable. However, there are things you can do to attain optimum wellness. Getting proper medical care, good nutrition, and adequate sleep and rest; keeping physically fit; and avoiding things that may trigger a seizure can help you live a healthier life. Additional support and information are available from the Epilepsy Foundation of America, which is listed in the Resources section at the end of this book.

PART THREE

MENTAL ASPECTS

INTRODUCTION

Seven years ago, Valerie writes, she was "still me." At that time, she was concentrating on helping her husband, a native of Italy who was not yet very proficient in English, to set up a business. Only a quarter-mile from her home in Maryland, Valerie's car was struck by a vehicle whose driver wasn't looking as he pulled out into the road. Valerie was thrown down across the bench seat of her car. She recalls opening her eyes and finding herself on the floor—she was unaware of having struck her head, but remembers experiencing a flash of tremendous rage. Disoriented and shaky, but with no specific complaints, Valerie was driven home.

The next day, Valerie went to the emergency room because she couldn't see straight and felt very confused. The doctor diagnosed a concussion with some muscle strain but took no x-rays. Four days later, a general practitioner prescribed Darvocet, a powerful painkiller, and amitriptyline, an antidepressant used as a painkiller. The medications put Valerie in such a fog that she threw them out a week or two later.

Valerie remembers little about the first year and a half after her accident, but recalls seing a neurologist who diagnosed postconcussive syndrome, and told her that her symptoms would disappear in three to six months. Her MRI and CT scan results were normal. However, for two and a half years after her MTBI, and occasionally even today, people around Valerie can see her eyes glaze over when lights, noise, or too much information causes sensory overload. Currently, Valerie has trouble remembering what she has just said or done, and she cannot recall the past except in bits and pieces. Her ability to concentrate and follow through is very limited, as is her ability to organize, prioritize, and initiate activities. Her depth perception and visual tracking are impaired, which causes all sorts of dyslexic phenomena, and she has problems with eye-hand coordination. Valerie's MTBI also has a strong emotional component that includes irritability, mood swings, and self-doubt—especially concerning memory and judgment.

The thinking process involves a number of different components, including how you register information through attention and concentration; how you store and retrieve incoming messages; and how you reason, plan, organize, initiate, comprehend, learn new information, and create new ideas. It also involves your ability to understand language, read and write, and do mathematics.

Many people with MTBI encounter a variety of mental effects in the months and years after injury. Part Three of this book considers the different aspects of your thinking abililty and provides information about mental difficulties frequently associated with MTBI, along with information about diagnosis and treatment and practical suggestions that can help minimize the effects of such problems.

13

ATTENTION AND CONCENTRATION

After suffering an MTBI, Gail, whose story appears in Chapter 4, struggled with sensory overload caused by her body's inability to regulate incoming sensations such as sound, light, and touch. She walked strangely, because she couldn't tolerate the sensation of her feet touching the ground. If someone touched her elbow, she would jump backward. Previously, ordinary night sounds had been soothing; now they caused Gail to lie awake at night, listening to cars that sounded as if they were right outside the window, rather than on the highway a half-mile away. She was disturbed by the sounds of birds moving in the trees and crickets in the grass. Daytime noise was completely intolerable, as were bright, blinking, or fluorescent lights.

By the third year after her accident, Gail's regulating ability had improved markedly. She is now able to select which incoming sensation she wants to attend to and thus is better able to concentrate. She feels that this improvement is probably the result of conditioning herself to her increased awareness of sound and light. However, she still avoids shopping malls and other busy places.

Focusing your attention and concentrating are automatic, spontaneous processes of registering information from sensory and other input. In general, problems in this area go unnoticed until some incident causes you to take notice—for instance, a pot boiling over on the stove. And even these situations are usually chalked up to a faulty memory, rather than to problems with attention.

After an MTBI, attention and concentration problems may occur more frequently than before, and your lack of awareness may disrupt your ability to work, maintain social connections, carry out various tasks, or tend to personal matters. A problem like Gail's—an inability to select or filter incoming sensations—can cause actual discomfort, as well as difficulty concentrating. While it can be hard to live with sudden distractibility or overattentiveness, understanding the nature of your problem and developing a set of management techniques can help immensely.

WHY ATTENTION AND CONCENTRATION PROBLEMS CAN OCCUR AFTER MTBI

Attention is the ability to focus on specific messages; *concentration* is the capacity to maintain attention to that message. These abilities enable you to select which input from bodily sensations and your surrounding environment you wish to respond to, as well as to shift from one activity or thought to another. It is believed that damage to the upper brain stem and frontal lobes (see Chapter 1), or diffuse damage to the body's connections to these areas, can cause permanent changes in your ability to attend to and register messages from your body and the outside world.

WHAT MTBI-RELATED ATTENTION AND CONCENTRATION PROBLEMS ARE LIKE

"Because of sensory overload problems after my MTBI, it took me five years to become able to dine in a restaurant or attend a carnival again. Before, I would become physically ill and feel as if I were about to pass out. At home, I had to eliminate background noise before I answered the phone so that I could attend to what was being said. I also needed complete silence when I was writing or working on the computer. To exercise my ability to focus and concentrate, I used the solitaire game that came with my computer program. In addition, my family helped me to make lists for shopping and daily routines, which I stored in the computer and retrieved as needed. It was not until I did a year of EEG biofeedback in my seventh year of recovery that my attention and concentration problems showed marked improvement."

—D.R.S.

Like many brain functions, attention and concentration are dynamic and complex operations. They have three main components—alertness; capacity for and sustained attention; and selection. An MTBI can affect any or all of these.

Alertness

Alertness is the general readiness that enables you to act upon information from your surroundings, such as sounds, movements, or events.

For example, it is alertness that creates an awareness that the phone is ringing or that a mosquito has bitten you. Sleep problems, which often result from MTBI, frequently cause problems with alertness and awareness. Fatigue, medication, depression, anxiety, and the consumption of alcohol can also dramatically diminish your alertness level—sometimes to the point that incoming information is never registered.

Capacity for and Sustained Attention

Your capacity for attention is the amount of information you are able to take in and process at a given moment. For instance, most people can receive and mentally hold on to a seven-digit telephone number long enough to write it down.

Sustained attention refers to the ability to focus and concentrate on a task or thought for a period of time while filtering out other information from your body or from the environment. After a brain injury, you may find concentrating extremely difficult due to fatigue, distractibility, or the fact that you cannot stop your mind from wandering. You may encounter problems with reading, following directions, or even holding a conversation. Also, you may find that you can concentrate on certain things—phone calls, for instance—only at particular times of the day.

Selection

"On a walk with my husband, I was nearly hit by an oncoming car. My husband yelled at me for not moving aside, but in that moment, he forgot that I had problems with attention and selection. Of course I saw the car, but since information I perceive isn't always registered properly, I didn't respond."
—D.R.S.

The capacity to choose what you wish to concentrate on is referred to as *selection*. This ability includes all of your senses and occurs spontaneously. Selection has two main parts—*filtering*, or selecting an experience to focus on, and *shifting*, or moving your attention from one experience to another. Filtering is what allows you to concentrate on reading the newspaper despite a fly buzzing around you and the noise of neighborhood children at play. If your ability to filter has been affected by your MTBI, you can be impervious to things you should notice or overwhelmed by normal background sounds and distractions. *Overfiltering* can affect your general alertness and awareness of danger signals or distractions, while *underfiltering* can disrupt your ability to focus. In either case, the result is difficulty completing any task.

Shifting is what allows you to quickly transfer your attention from the magazine article you are reading to a friend calling your name from another room. Problems with shifting ability can cause you to repeat thoughts over and over, or to linger on a topic or problem long after others have lost interest. This particular symptom of shifting problems is called *perseveration*.

Filtering and shifting problems can combine to create sensory overload, which most commonly affects the senses of hearing and sight. Hearing overload can cause sounds to be magnified or make it difficult to understand conversation in a noisy room. Visual overload creates sensitivity to light, especially the fluorescent lighting used in many offices, stores, and other public places. Sensory overload can result in mental fatigue as your mind tries to make sense of all the incoming information. Factors that can contribute to sensory overload include medications, caffeine, hormonal changes, and attention deficit disorders.

DIAGNOSING ATTENTION AND CONCENTRATION PROBLEMS

Diagnosing attention and concentration problems can be difficult, because each MTBI is unique. You may experience one or a combination of attention problems. Whatever your complaint, you may undergo both formal standardized testing and informal assessments.

A thorough neurological examination and neuropsychological testing should be done to determine your ability to attend to messages, tasks, and situations, and to establish a baseline against which subsequent improvement can be measured. In particular, neuropsychological testing—which compares your current level of functioning to your prior capabilities—can yield important information about specific deficits and possible treatments.

Other types of standardized testing may also be done. Tests measuring arousal responses—heart rate, skin temperature, muscle tension, and brain activity—are available but may not be necessary, because most people with MTBI can report how they feel or how they perform at school, work, and home. If your responses differ depending on your environment, response testing can pinpoint situations that trigger problems. Tests for sensory overload can be done by an appropriate specialist, such as an audiologist, who can administer an evaluation and central auditory process test to measure your hearing ability and your capacity for attending to sound.

Informal testing, in the form of simple observations of your functioning, may be done at home, at work, or in the classroom. These informal assessments can take the form of behavioral scales or checklists that contain lists of symptoms to be rated on a frequency scale of 0 to 5. You, or a professional observer, would be asked to assign a frequency to such items as your ability to understand conversation in a crowded room. Informal testing helps to determine how often and under what circumstances you miss being aware of information, become distracted, or experience sensory overload. These assessments help evaluate the character or quality of stimuli or activities that cause you to respond—for example, whether you respond to the intensity of the sound of a clock alarm, or to the duration of the sound.

It can also be very helpful to keep a log recording your difficulties with selection, concentration, or alertness. This will help you to identify and understand the circumstances that pose problems.

TREATING MTBI-RELATED ATTENTION AND CONCENTRATION PROBLEMS

The results of both formal and informal assessments help with the development of a treatment plan pinpointing such things as situations that you should avoid and the best times of day for you to perform problem activities. Naturally, you will want to play an active role in designing a treatment program for your attention and concentration problems. If focusing difficulties sometimes cause you to miss parts of conversations, you may wish to audiotape your discussions of test results with your neurologist or neuropsychologist.

Proper diagnosis will permit your specialist to identify very specific problem areas—for instance, problems filtering out distracting sounds or movement. There are specific rehabilitation programs available that offer retraining or teach you ways to compensate for such deficits. Your neurologist, neuropsychologist, or local hospital should be able to help you locate a program in your area. Your doctor can also suggest and, if necessary, teach you the treatment methods discussed below.

Conventional Approaches

The type of treatment appropriate for attention and concentration problems is as unique as each person who experiences MTBI. It is important that the methods and techniques developed for you be matched to your requirements. Based on what has been learned through testing and your own observations, you should have some idea of the types of situations that cause problems, and you will probably want to simply avoid them as much as possible, at least for the time being. Cognitive-behavioral therapy can help you to control your environment and/or to learn ways of coping with those things that cannot be changed or avoided. For example, you may learn to regulate the times of day that you go outdoors. Or you may discover that certain colors cause sensory overload and that simply repainting the walls of your home minimizes the problem.

EEG biofeedback, which trains the brain to increase alert, or beta, waves while decreasing slower theta waves, has been found to be extremely effective for attention disorders. Hypnosis is also frequently used to help people with MTBI learn to modify their perception of or reactions to stimuli. Certain medications, such as methylphenidate (Ritalin) and dextroamphetamine (Dexedrine), can be very effective for attention problems. You may also be able to receive tutoring and additional help from a learning-disabilities specialist. Your local school district should be able to put you in touch with a teacher trained in working with people with attention deficit difficulties.

The process of identifying specific problems and making appropriate changes is not easy. It can take months just to pin down symptoms and triggers. But with patience, and with the guidance of understanding professionals, you are sure to see progress.

Alternative Approaches

Polarity therapy may be helpful in resolving attention and concentration problems, particularly if the practitioner has experience treating your particular symptoms.

Ginkgo biloba, ginseng, super blue-green algae, black cohosh, and suan zoa ren are among herbal preparations sometimes cited as beneficial for mental functioning. Remedies that may be suggested by homeopaths for these problems include *Phosphoricum acidum*, *Helleborus*, and *Calcaria carbonica*. We recommend that you seek the advice of a qualified herbalist or homeopath who has experience in MTBI, rather than experimenting with over-the-counter products on your own. If your physician is unable to provide an appropriate referral, an organization such as the Herb Research Foundation or the National Center for Homeopathy (see the Resources section beginning on page 281) may be able to help.

PRACTICAL SUGGESTIONS

"I always carry earplugs and sunglasses to use at the first sign of sensory overload. I also find a baseball cap helpful for reducing overhead stimuli when I shop or travel. In public places, I walk close to walls and keep my atten-

tion focused away from crowds. If I am with someone, I walk directly behind them or just slightly to the side so I can focus on the person's feet or back. To go grocery shopping, I make a list of the items I need in the order in which they are shelved in the store. I also select a quiet place to retreat to when I begin to feel overwhelmed. Most important, I try to stay sensitive to the signs of overload, since the problem is easier to handle in its early stages."

—Dena

"I space out tasks that tend to produce overload over the course of the day instead of trying to complete such jobs all at once. I also monitor those senses that are are most likely to overload so that overuse doesn't trigger problems."

—Judith

Getting proper rest and regular exercise, avoiding alcohol and drugs (except for those prescribed by your physician), and reducing the stress in your life are the first steps to take in overcoming problems with attention and concentration. Also, it is important to seek relief from postinjury pain, which in itself can be extremely distracting. At home and work, there are a number of commonsense ways to improve your ability to attend and concentrate. We have divided these into four groups: environmental modifications, time modifications, task modifications, and social modifications.

Environmental Modifications

When dealing with attention or concentration difficulties, environmental stimuli can play a major role. The following measures can help you to function at your best:

- When working or studying, do so in complete quiet. Keep the radio and the television *off* whenever you are attempting to focus on an activity. Turn off the ringer on your telephone and let an answering machine take your calls or, if necessary, look into hiring an answering service.

- Consider the lighting, furnishings, seating arrangements, ventilation, visual displays, and colors of your home and workplace carefully, with an eye toward eliminating sensory overload.

- Remove all nonessentials from bathroom and kitchen countertops. Keep necessary items in clearly marked different-colored containers.

- Use a telephone headset to keep your hands free and help focus your attention during calls.

If your environment interferes with your ability to concentrate on a task, it is reassuring to identify and, to the extent that this is possible, to avoid or change those aspects that trouble you most.

Time Modifications

It is not uncommon for people with MTBI to have fairly predictable daily patterns—specifically, good and bad times of day for focusing and maintaining attention. Recognizing and seeking to work within these patterns is one way of coping with the aftereffects of your injury. The following are a few suggestions:

- Keep a log of times and circumstances when you begin to lose your ability to concentrate, and adjust your schedule of activities accordingly.

- Take note of the time of day you perform different tasks, and observe how long it takes you to complete them. You may discover that you perform certain activities better at certain times of day.

- Watch closely for tiredness. Take frequent work or study breaks, varying the length of these interruptions. Notice how often and for how long you need to take breathers, and then institute a regular practice of doing so.

- Do what you can to remove time pressures. Minimize stress by allowing twice the time you think you will need to complete any task.

Everyone has times of day when he or she feels most alert. You will find concentrating easier once you begin planning your work activities accordingly.

Task Modifications

After an MTBI, it may be necessary to modify certain tasks—even the most basic and familiar—to compensate for deficits in attention and concentration. The following are suggestions that may help:

- Set realistic goals for performing tasks that require attention and concentration.

- Talk aloud as a reminder about coping strategies—for instance, ways to focus on conversation at a party or avoid commotions while shopping.

- Experiment with different ways of paying attention, but avoid added stress by giving yourself permission to fail.

- Investigate computer software programs designed to help with attention and concentration. These are most often created for children, but they can be helpful for adults with attention deficits as well. Microsoft has a DOS game called BOA that encourages focus, eye-hand coordination, and the ability to think quickly. The Learning Company offers others, such as Midnight Explorer, that yield similar results but are more complex.

- Practice focusing your attention with card games such as Concentration, a matching game that exercises both attention and concentration.

- Try coloring, an activity that forces you to focus on shape, color, and eye-hand coordination. Puzzles, knitting, and handcrafts require similar concentration.

- Improve your ability to focus when listening by having a friend or family member read aloud to you. Books on tape, available at most public libraries, can also help.

- Don't rush through tasks or expect a perfect performance.

For most people, the ability to attend and concentrate varies at times. If you have a pressing work or home project, the above suggestions can help.

Social Modifications

Problems with attention and concentration can affect every aspect of your life, including your social interactions. The following are a number of suggestions that can help you to cope with these new difficulties:

- Ask people to speak slowly when they dispense important information, giving a small bit of information at a time and pausing occasionally so you can process what they are saying. Do not hesitate to ask people to rephrase or repeat their statements if necessary. Afterwards, repeat or paraphrase what you have heard to ensure that you have the correct information.

- Take notes about what is being said, if necessary, or use a pocket tape recorder. Some are voice-activated and have small projection microphones, so they are not noticeable.

- Be honest and matter-of-fact about your attention and concentration problems. Doing so will help both you and the person you are speaking with feel more at ease.

• If your mind wanders when someone is speaking, try focusing on his or her voice quality or gestures.

Attention and concentration problems that follow MTBI can be disruptive and distressing. However, some of these difficulties diminish over time, and others respond well to treatment approaches that your specialist can recommend, as well as to practical coping techniques. Over time, you will likely discover at least some effective coping methods on your own. As with many other MTBI-related symptoms, time and support are your best allies.

14

MEMORY

Fifty-one-year-old Gracia was academic and executive director of a nonprofit organization. On her way home from work one February day, her car was sideswiped by a vehicle that had run a red light. Her car spun around 180 degrees before coming to a stop. Gracia was taken to the emergency room, where she was diagnosed with a mild concussion and sent home. At work the following day, she experienced a severe headache and dizziness. She also felt confused and couldn't figure out why she wasn't able to perform routine tasks.

Days later, Gracia returned to her doctor and underwent a battery of tests, including a skull x-ray, an MRI, a CT scan, and an EEG. All the test results were negative, but Gracia knew that something was drastically wrong. She asked for neuropsychological testing, but even this turned up no measurable brain damage.

Over a year later, Gracia was still unable to return to work. She was plagued by headaches, dizziness, extreme fatigue, confusion, and severe short-term memory problems. At times, she couldn't find the research library—a place she had visited several times a week for years. Other times, she would find herself outside the grocery store, unsure of where she was or how to get home. Sometimes Gracia was sure she was losing her mind.

The ability to store and recall information serves as one of the major criteria for determining the severity of brain injury. Memory problems are the most common and persistent of all neurological consequences of MTBI, and symptoms can vary from person to person. The types of memory problems that can result from MTBI include more than simple forgetfulness. They can involve the inability to recall events or to digest new information and ideas. The way you remember is also influenced by factors such as attention, organization, motivation, and fatigue, any or all of which may be affected by brain injury as well.

WHY MEMORY PROBLEMS CAN OCCUR AFTER MTBI

The processes involved in memory are very complex. Your memory is actually a number of interrelated networks for storing and retrieving information. This system allows you to store and recall simple sensory information as well as complex knowledge and personal experiences. Damage to any part of this intricate system can disrupt your ability to categorize, link, and recall recent thoughts and experiences. In turn, if you become unable to recall information, it can become extremely difficult to formulate new ideas or even to act upon old ones.

MTBI-related memory problems are believed to result from injury to the front or rear portions of the brain's frontal lobes, or to specific areas within the temporal lobes and to internal structures such as the hippocampus and amygdala (see Chapter 1). On occasion, the parietal lobes may be involved as well. Memory problems resulting from brain trauma can vary widely in nature and extent, depending on the site, complexity, and severity of the injury.

WHAT MTBI-RELATED MEMORY PROBLEMS ARE LIKE

"Each of my three sons has a different activity schedule. At times, because of my memory problems, I've literally lost my children. To help with this problem, I have learned to write down their schedules, along with when and where to pick them up. However, there have been a few times when I've forgotten where I placed the written schedule and was unable to recall where my sons were. Naturally, this terrifies me."

—D.R.S.

The processes of forming and retrieving memories are complex, involving three distinct phases: registration, storage, and retrieval. The types of memory problems that result from any individual MTBI depend on which of these are affected.

Registration

Registration, also called *encoding,* involves the perception of environmental information and sensory input. Sensory impairment, such as that which can result from MTBI, can affect how—or whether—certain environmental messages are perceived. Attention problems (see Chapter 13) also can interfere with the amount of information you are able to register, and the accuracy with which you can do so.

Storage

"I can recall everything prior to my MTBI, but have no memory of the accident itself and now have great difficulty learning and remembering new information. It feels strange to recall certain parts of events so vividly and have absolutely no memory of other parts. When this happens, even hints and cues fail to evoke recall of the incident. It's as if there are huge holes or gaps in my memory."

—D.R.S.

The second phase of memory is *storage*. How you store information is the key to a keen memory. Studies show that relating new material to previously learned information helps to form new pathways between the cells of the brain for more efficient storage of information. There are three types of memory storage: sensory memory, short-term memory, and long-term memory.

Sensory memory is the storage of information that lasts only seconds but leaves a lingering sight, smell, sound, or sensation, such as when a fly brushes against your skin. This type of memory works hand in hand with attention. If you cannot recall the name of someone you were just introduced to, or you cannot recall the phone number just recited by the operator, it is usually inattention that has prevented the information from being stored. However, if you have deficits affecting sensory memory, you may be unable to play back in your mind what you have just heard. In the case of visual images, you may be unable to picture a bit of information. Deficits in sensory memory often go unnoticed. After all, if you don't notice something in the first place, you cannot be aware of not remembering it.

Short-term memory, also called *buffer memory* or *working memory*, is the part of the memory process that receives and recalls chunks of information for up to one minute. Short-term memory is what enables you to integrate previously learned information with new information to form creative or novel thoughts. It is critical to daily living; it is what makes it possible for you to recall where you placed your car keys or checkbook, whether you locked the door or turned off the stove, and whether you have eaten or bathed. In the best of circumstances, short-term memory has a limited storage capacity. This type of memory is the most susceptible to interference from the pain, stress, fatigue, attention problems, and sensory overload that can follow MTBI. For example, if you are interrupted while receiving a bit of information, the thought may be lost.

Long-term memory, also called *remote* or *secondary memory,* differs from short-term memory in duration, capacity, and manner of storage. Long-term memories are information received and held beyond one minute, becoming learned information. Research suggests that the capacity of long-term memory is immeasurable, in contrast to short-term memory's limited capacity, and that the reliving or reexperiencing of memories solidifies their place in long-term storage. After MTBI, long-term memories tend to return in fits and starts. Some may never be fully recovered. In some cases, whole areas of information are lost while related information remains intact. For instance, you may be able to recall that George Washington was the first president of the United States, but be unable to recall anything about Abraham Lincoln, even with prompting. This type of long-term memory loss is called the "Swiss-cheese effect."

Usually, after an MTBI, long-past memories are the easiest to access, followed by events closer in time to the injury. Verbal memory problems and word-finding deficits can continue for years. Following an MTBI, learning new material—which requires attention, organization, and sensory and short-term memory—is often extremely difficult. A common sign of a long-term memory problem is a vague sense that you are reliving a thought or situation, often called *déjà vu.* After MTBI, this may occur because you are unaware that you are actually recalling a past experience.

Retrieval

The last phase of memory is *retrieval,* your ability to access stored information. Retrieval can occur only if both registration and storage have taken place. It is based on cues that trigger your memory of how the information was first registered. Smells, sights, sounds, and emotions, for example, are often linked to memories; this is why hearing an old song can momentarily take you back to the past.

Research shows that information is more easily accessed if you can reproduce the state in which it was registered, either physically or through hypnosis. Any form of stress, fatigue, anxiety, or depression can interfere with this ability. Memory-retrieval problems can range from "tip-of-the-tongue" struggles, to an inability to describe a missing word or thought, to amnesia, or complete inability to access information. Or other thoughts may intrude, information may be recalled incorrectly, or messages may be lost among other information.

Forgetting occurs when a particular memory is not accessible. This can mean that the information is no longer stored, or that there is some sort of internal or external interference with the memory. Often, forgetting results from poor organization of information to be stored. For instance, if someone tells you his or her phone number, you need to repeat the number or link it with other information, such as the year you were born or some other familiar number, in order to remember it. Without this step of practice, the information is more likely to be lost. Other considerations in the proper storage and retrieval of information include emotions and psychological factors; the use of certain drugs, including a number of prescription medications as well as alcohol and recreational drugs; and auditory or visual distractions.

Many people with MTBI experience problems with the registration or storage of messages. However, you may not become aware that you have a memory problem until you try to retrieve information at some later point and find you are unable to do so.

Problems with amnesia, or total absence of recall, can also occur following MTBI. There are different types of amnesia. *Retrograde amnesia* affects the ability to recall events prior to a traumatic event—in this case, an MTBI. At times, you may recall bits and pieces of certain events, but other memories remain absent. Specific brain functions such as sensory and motor abilities can also be affected. *Anterograde amnesia*, sometimes called *posttraumatic amnesia,* affects the ability to remember events following MTBI or other traumatic event. Neither *total amnesia,* the complete loss of memory, nor *psychogenic amnesia,* a dissociative disorder, is commonly associated with MTBI. (A detailed discussion of dissociative disorders will be found in Chapter 20.)

DIAGNOSING MEMORY PROBLEMS

A thorough neuropsychological evaluation is the best way to evaluate memory problems. This assessment compares your present level of functioning with your previous abilities (see Chapter 2). From this battery of diagnostic tests, an appropriate treatment plan can be developed, so it is vital that your neurospychologist explain your results in detail.

TREATING MTBI-RELATED MEMORY PROBLEMS

"When learning new things, I repeat information or write it down over and over until I am able to recall it. New piano pieces are a particular struggle; however, if I record the music on a variable-speed tape recorder, I can practice troublesome sections over and over until I get them right. In my work as a psychologist, I repeat or paraphrase what my patients tell me and im-

mediately write down cues to what is meant. A pocket-sized memo recorder, which holds up to five messages, is also very helpful. Computer games and programs have helped me to sequence and recall information."

—D.R.S.

The appropriate treatment for memory problems depends on the source of the difficulty. If testing determines that you are experiencing problems remembering things because of a failure to register information properly, you will need to focus on improving your ability to direct and maintain your attention (Chapter 13 presents treatment suggestions and practical tips that can help). If you are affected by amnesia, time without stress is the best antidote. Short- and long-term memory problems respond to various approaches, the most common of which are described below.

Conventional Approaches

Time often heals memory loss. Long-term memory loss may be helped with hypnosis, which can be effective at retreiving past memories. Impaired short-term memory function may respond to treatment with certain medications, including methylphenidate (Ritalin), a stimulant that can be helpful for attention disorders, and amantadine (Symmetrel), a drug that affects the action of brain chemicals called neurotransmitters and that is sometimes used to treat people with Parkinson's disease. These medications have side effects, but if they are effective, the benefits may outweigh the disadvantages.

Rehabilitation centers often offer programs to help you manage persistent memory problems. One approach is to help you reacquire or improve lost skills through training or tutoring. Another approach is *compensatory intervention,* which teaches you to work around your deficits by learning alternative ways to accomplish specific tasks or behaviors. You are taught how to use your present skills and your innate learning style to recall information. Internal cues such as sensations and thoughts, as well as external cues like color or sound, may be used. The Brain Injury Association (see the Resources section at the end of this book) can refer you to a center in your area that provides compensatory memory training.

Alternative Approaches

Many advertisements state that certain herbs or homeopathic remedies can increase your memory. These over-the-counter products may help, but it is always best to work with a knowledgeable practitioner rather than attempting to self-medicate. Even natural remedies can have serious side effects if not used properly. Depending on your specific needs, a knowledgeable herbalist may recommend a product such as ginkgo biloba, ginseng, super blue-green algae, black cohosh, or suan zoa ren for memory improvement. Homeopathic remedies that may be recommended for people with MTBI-related memory difficulties include *Carbo vegetabilis, Silicea terra,* and *Hyoscyamus niger.* If your physician is unable to help you with herbs and/or homeopathics or to provide a referral to a practitioner who can, the Herb Research Foundation and/or the National Center for Homeopathy (see the Resources Section beginning on page 281) can help you locate an appropriate practitioner in your area.

Some people have found that taking certain nutritional supplements, such as 50 milligrams of vitamin B_6 (pyridoxine) and 100 milligrams of coenzyme Q_{10} daily, have helped to restore memory. It is important to be aware, however, that excessive amounts of vitamin B_6 can damage the nervous system. As with any substance, it is crucial to first confer with your physician to determine what dosage, if any, is best for you.

PRACTICAL SUGGESTIONS

"I suffered an MTBI after winning a $30,000 academic scholarship, and began to find answering multiple-part questions to be a problem due to short-term memory limitations. Now, each time someone asks me a two-part question, I subtly touch a fingertip to the table and leave it there as a signal to myself. I answer the first question, then casually say, "Now, what was the second part of your question?" Once the second question is answered, I remove my hand from the table."

—Julia

"I find I remember things better with lots of practice. I provide three or four friends with a list of possible questions about material I am committing to memory and ask them to grill me on the information."

—Don

It takes a tremendous amount of energy to think clearly. Extensive periods of thinking and concentrating can cause mental fatigue under the best of circumstances, and will certainly do so in the aftermath of an MTBI. Often, a vicious cycle results as you struggle to remember something, discover that you cannot, and then feel even more exhausted.

It is important to bear your new limitations in mind, but equally important not to let your symptoms defeat you. The following are some strategies that can help you register, store, and recall information more efficiently:

- Restrict your use of alcohol. Drinking has a direct effect on memory and cognition. Not only that, but your MTBI may have reduced your tolerance.

- Ask your doctor if one or more of the medications you take may be causing short-term memory loss as a side effect. If so, discuss whether the benefits of the medication outweigh the effects on your ability to remember.

- Have clocks and calendars visible around the house, especially in your bedroom and work areas.

- Categorize and group incoming information in small, concise pieces such as work-related details, tasks to be done, and phone calls to be made.

- Color-code objects by category or event at home and work by giving each week a specific color. Using appropriately colored stickers can help you recall which week a project is to be done, or what week you purchased certain food items. A friend or family member can help you reorganize things.

- Visualize details of your destination and how to get there before leaving home.

- Close your eyes after you set down an item such as your glasses or keys, and picture in your mind where you have placed it. Then open your eyes and look again to reinforce this image. If you are a tactile person, touch the area; if you use scents as cues, smell the area; and if you are a verbal person, say aloud what you see.

- Make it a practice to finish one task before beginning another. This way, you don't have to to remember where you stopped. If this is impossible, use color tags, book markers, or notes to yourself as reminders of where you stopped in your projects. A task log can be very helpful.

- Play card games such as Concentration and Memory. These matching games help with attention, concentration, and recall.

- Do memory exercises. For example, have a friend or family member show you pictures, then put the pictures aside and ask you to identify what you saw. Audio programs such as Kevin Trudeau's

Mega Memory from Cybervision provide a step-by-step course in improving your memory. Computer programs such as Challenge of the Ancients from The Learning Company are designed for fun but can improve your ability to recall things.

- Experiment to determine your stronger points, memory-wise, and use your strengths to help you recall things. For example, if your visual channel is impaired and you have trouble remembering things you have seen, try touching or smelling things to aid you in creating memory more effectively.

- Use tone and rhythm cues to help you store and recall information. By listening you may be able to store such information as the fact that you vacuumed the living room (a muffled sound) not the kitchen (a sharper sound), or that glasses, not paper cups, go in the dishwasher.

- Consider using a device such as a pocket computer, voice-activated tape recorder, notebook computer, or daily planner to help you keep track of important information.

- Use initial consonants and silly stories, songs, and acronyms to trigger auditory memories, just as advertisers do. For example, you might chant or sing "hat-hamp" to remind yourself to get the hat near the hamper, or "OJ" to remember to buy orange juice at the store.

- Put different scents on different objects to stimulate your olfactory memory—the very first memory used in life. Read up on aromatherapy and explore the different scents that can enhance your recall.

- Distinguish work or school materials by covering them in different textures or fabrics. Touch is the second sensory memory used in life, and different surfaces can serve as memory cues.

- Post notes, signs, and checklists to remind yourself what to do and when. A list on the front door can help you remember to turn off the coffeepot and take your keys, while a note on the bathroom mirror can remind you to floss your teeth before you go to bed at night.

- Decide on proper places for items such as your keys, glasses, wallet, or wristwatch, and be certain always to place things where they belong. If necessary, compile a master list of objects and their locations and store copies around your house and on your computer, if you have one.

At best, memory problems are quite frustrating. At worst, they are distressing. Time may eventually heal your recall problems, but devising strategies that employ your personal style of learning and experimenting with different approaches and techniques can help you cope in the meantime.

15

REASONING, PLANNING, AND UNDERSTANDING

Barbara was a sixth-grade teacher in Massachusetts. At school one day, a student dropped a basketball down a stairwell. Barbara, who was standing on a lower staircase, was hit on the head and knocked unconscious. She then fell down the flight of stairs. Afterward, Barbara regained consciousness and looked and sounded fine; however, she soon realized that something was very wrong. For instance, she could no longer take care of bill-paying. Ashamed to admit this, she hid months' worth of bills—a fact her family discovered only when their power was shut off. Then Barbara was unable to find the bills she had hidden. Once a highly organized teacher, she found herself similarly unable to function in the classroom, although for a long time she didn't understand why she couldn't work. She simply couldn't judge the extent of her brain injury.

Aside from organizational, memory, and task-management problems, Barbara has serious trouble with the concept of time. She no longer understands or relates to the passage of minutes, hours, or days. Her old routines are currently impossible, though Barbara has learned to set timers all around her house to help her plan and follow a simple daily itinerary.

Rarely do we stop to consider how it is that we think, for doing so is as automatic as the beating of one's heart. After an MTBI, however, even simple tasks can require a great deal of thought, leading people who are unaware of what has happened to suddenly feel incapable or stupid. Activities that require so-called *executive functions*—that is, the ability to reason, make sound judgments, and initiate, plan, or organize—may become virtually impossible, and this can pose a serious threat to independent living.

WHY EXECUTIVE FUNCTION PROBLEMS CAN OCCUR AFTER MTBI

Problems associated with planning, organizing, initiating, making sound judgments, and understanding are often linked to injury to the brain's frontal lobes (see Chapter 1). However, research suggests that executive functions are complex processes involving several brain areas. Therefore, it is generalized rather than localized brain trauma that is responsible for post-MTBI problems with executive functions. Fortunately, the complete loss of executive function following this type of injury is rare.

TYPES OF EXECUTIVE FUNCTION PROBLEMS THAT CAN FOLLOW MTBI

"The first time I became aware of my reasoning problems was six months after my accident. We were packing for a trip to the mountains, and my husband suggested that I set out the clothing I needed. A while later, he found me crying, for I had no idea what to do or what to pack. Up to that time, we hadn't truly comprehended the extent of my limitations."

—D.R.S.

The ability to reason and think is not a single process, but an extremely complex network of related processes. Each of the abilities that make up your executive functions depends upon other mental processes to enable you to receive, comprehend, and act appropriately upon information. A problem with any one area can affect your overall thinking ability, just as a problem with one small part of the engine can affect the overall operation of your car. The following are descriptions of some of the higher-level thinking problems that commonly follow MTBI.

Planning

The ability to plan is the capacity for thinking ahead and setting goals, whether for the next hour, the next week, or the next year. Planning is the first step in organizing daily living—you must decide what it is you want to do before you can determine how to accomplish it. Impaired planning ability undermines your ability to set goals, so if you suffer from this problem, you may need to rely on others to make plans for you, or play it safe by avoiding anything other than a repetetive routine.

Organization

"A year and a half after my accident, my husband, believing that I was much better, invited guests for a Fourth-of-July barbecue. Prior to my MTBI, such parties were common events at our house. Now, however, I had no idea what a barbecue was or how to organize one. Happily, this problem has since improved greatly."

—D.R.S.

Organization is the ability to determine how your daily plans are going to be accomplished. For instance, if you are planning dinner, you must first decide what foods will be included, whether you need to take anything out of the freezer, whether a trip to the store is required, and when to start preparing each of the different dishes included in the meal so that they are all ready at the same time. Together, planning and organizing require skills in concentration, memory, problem-solving, and sequencing (putting or recalling events in order, or breaking a task into necessary steps). If you have problems with organization, you may encounter difficulty giving directions or breaking down a task. If you cannot track and sequence the past, present, and future, it will seem as if time has been altered or become nonexistent—as if you have somehow lost time. Often, the emotional result is a general feeling of anxiety, which can further impair your ability to organize, as well as aggravating your MTBI symptoms in general.

Initiation

Initiation is the ability to carry out the tasks you have set for yourself—the ability to translate thoughts into activity. Even if you are able to plan and organize, an MTBI may leave you unable to initiate the actions you have planned. To family and friends, this can look like a motivational problem, but an inability to initiate is in fact unrelated to energy level or ambition. Rather, the injury may have left your brain unable to take even the most specific and detailed thought and turn it into activity.

Processing Information

This phase of executive function is the lightning-quick combination of a multitude of new pieces of sensory information with existing knowledge. An MTBI can affect the speed, duration, and accuracy of the integration, and later interpretation, of such input. Such a processing delay can cost you precious minutes in reaction time, perhaps leading to injury. For instance, you might not know to immediately remove your finger from a hot stovetop if there is a delay or other problem in processing the incoming signal of heat. Or a clear message may lead to an inappropriate response, such as yelling "Fire!" in a crowded theater and then wondering why you are in the middle of a riot.

Comprehension

Comprehension is the ability to make sense out of processed and registered information—for instance, grasping the meaning of subtle humor or a complex story line in a movie. After MTBI, you may miss these messages. You may also be unable to understand verbal directions, commands, or questions, and be unable to make sense of maps and signs. In extreme cases, this problem can take the form of visual agnosia—the inability to recognize familiar objects or surroundings—causing the person with MTBI to get lost inside his or her own home or become unable to recognize family members.

Decision-Making

Even mild problems making judgments and decisions can affect all aspects of your thinking. Everyday activities such as cooking, shopping, or driving may suddenly become impossible if you ponder at length what used to be split-second decisions—such as knowing not to order an item you already own from a telemarketing salesperson. After an MTBI, you may find yourself making business decisions that you later regret. Judgment problems stem from four sources: awareness, selection, memory, and emotions. Obviously, if you have a problem with awareness, or attention, you may overlook information that is needed to make a sound decision, such as the cost of an item you are considering purchasing. If you cannot focus or remember, you will also have problems making choices that are appropriate. If you are upset or anxious, this too will interfere with your ability to make accurate and appropriate decisions.

Judgment difficulties range from mild to severe, and they affect concrete behavior, such as exercising caution at a stop sign, as well as higher-level problem-solving. Many MTBI people deny their decision-making problems at first for fear of appearing incompetent or stupid, but colleagues, family members, or friends often provide insight by pointing out gross errors in judgment.

Learning

After an MTBI, you may retain and use many of your old skills but be unable to acquire and use new information. For example, you may be extremely proficient at using a computer program you learned prior to your injury, but, despite weeks of training, fail to master even the basics of a new program. Even though you may not have any muscular or motor problems, you may also encounter difficulty learning new physical activities, such as a dance step or basketball move.

Creativity

Creativity is the process of developing new and original thoughts, plans, and solutions to problems. Researchers believe that the creative process begins in the right hemisphere of the brain. Of course, it is very difficult to form new ideas if your executive thinking skills have been impaired by an MTBI. You may misjudge the appropriateness or feasibility of an idea, or simply have trouble focusing on or remembering different facets of your thoughts. In addition, you may have trouble organizing and following through with the creative process, which means that you cannot act on novel ideas that do occur to you.

DIAGNOSING EXECUTIVE FUNCTION PROBLEMS

A thorough neuropsychological examination (see Chapter 2) is the best method of evaluating deficits in reasoning, planning, and understanding. This series of tests compares your current level of functioning with your previous abilities and can pinpoint specific problem areas. The results will enable you and the specialists involved in your care to develop a treatment program for your individual needs.

TREATING MTBI-RELATED EXECUTIVE FUNCTION PROBLEMS

"I have lost some of my sense of time. I never know how many minutes elapse when I'm talking to someone. I've learned over the years to watch the clock when talking and to ask friends to let me know when they have to hang up the phone. Also, as the mother of three teenagers, I do a lot of driving. I've learned to clock my trips ahead of time and write a schedule of places to be and the travel time involved. Preparing a schedule also enables me to ask for help recalling things or places I've forgotten."

—D.R.S.

Trusting others is the first step toward recovery from the reasoning, planning, and understanding problems that can surface after MTBI. It is important to allow friends and family members to help you, and to let go of the idea that you alone know what is best. The following are some approaches that your doctors may recommend.

Conventional Approaches

In many cases, executive function problems improve with time. At present, there are no medications known to help. While alcohol and recreational drugs may give a false sense of being able to think better, these substances actually interfere with healing and thought processes. Drugs and alcohol also contribute to fatigue and, in some cases, seizures.

Most rehabilitation hospitals offer treatment programs to help remediate deficits in executive functions. These programs help you develop skills to compensate for your inabilities, and teach you to use the skills you have retained more effectively. In general, five main areas are emphasized: awareness, goal formulation, planning and organization, initiation, and self-regulation (the ability to monitor your problems by yourself). You are taught how to identify problems and select solutions, and learn to review options and to sequence parts of a task. You are shown various compensatory strategies and trained to identify and correct errors in thinking and reasoning. In addition, you learn how to avoid distraction and effectively use support. Each MTBI is unique, but you and the rehabilitation staff will soon learn which techniques work best for you.

Alternative Approaches

There are a number of herbal and homeopathic products advertised that are supposed to help you think clearly and accurately. To determine what might be appropriate for your specific MTBI-related executive function problems, it is best to consult with an herbalist or homeopathic practitioner who is experienced in these areas. Your physician, the Herb Research Foundation, or the National Center for Homeopathy should be able to provide referrals to the type of practitioner or practitioners you need. An herbalist may suggest such products as ginkgo biloba, anise, blue cohosh, or chuaw xiong. The homeopathic remedies *Staphysagria, Phosphorus, Arnica,* and *Natrum sulphuricum* may also be recommended.

PRACTICAL SUGGESTIONS

"I use a digital watch to help with my awareness of time. Each 'beep' reminds me that another hour has passed, and the alarm feature helps keep me on time for appointments. On trips, I carry a timer as a supplement to my watch."

—*Patricia*

"My efforts to organize my home have concentrated in the kitchen. Lists of contents are posted on cabinet doors, and I keep a blueprint in a drawer for reference. My refrigerator and pantries are inventoried, and I update the list every time I remove or replace an item."

—Elizabeth

"I keep three different-colored book bags packed for school, and my husband reminds me of what day it is and which bag I need that day. I have an assistant who helps me to grade papers, and I color-code folders containing class notes, exercises, and exams before storing them in master folders labeled for each of my fifteen class sessions."

—Mary Beth

"I combat my reasoning and organization problems by carrying a DAY-TIMER appointment book and pen everywhere I go. I also write a task sheet outlining what needs to be done to start and finish each day, and I rely strongly on a watch with an hourly 'beep' and several alarms."

—Chris

If you have had an MTBI, you may face much more of a challenge as you go about your work and home life. It helps to take each day as it comes, accepting that your ability to reason, plan, understand, and learn new things may sometimes fluctuate. The following are some ways to minimize the disruption caused by executive function problems:

- Acknowledge that your brain has been damaged, and that this will affect your life. Accept the fact that learning new things, making appropriate judgments, and other tasks are now difficult for you, and remind yourself that mental disability is not the same thing as a lack of intelligence.

- Tell others of your need for quiet during work periods. If no distraction-free area exists at home, use a study carrel or reading room at your local public library.

- Discuss with your employer ways to provide you with a place in which you are able to do your work. This type of accommodation is required under the Americans With Disabilities Act.

- Check to see whether your insurance company will cover the cost of a home health aide to help with everyday tasks, such as meal preparation, that you are unable to do because of executive function problems.

- When your thoughts become disorganized, seek out a peaceful place. A church, park, or college campus can be an excellent place to "regroup."

- Build a support system to help you deal with daily frustrations. This can include therapists, your friends and family, a brain-injury support group, and/or an on-line bulletin board.

- Use a VCR or tape player to help you improve your ability to sequence sights and sounds. These devices allow you to repeat bits of information until you grasp the meaning of what is being presented.

- Use a timer to relieve anxiety about forgetting tasks or appointments and to help with time management.

- Make notes via tape recorder, daily planner, computer, or notebook to help with short-term memory, planning, and organizing problems.

- Ask someone else to take charge of bill-paying for the present. There are also computer programs, such as Quicken, that can help to guide you through this task.

- Allow more time than you think you will need to learn new tasks. Be patient, and deal only with today's problem.

- Be willing to put aside tasks that prove too difficult for now. Chances are, you will be able to learn (or relearn) needed skills later.

- Work at regaining your perception of time by noting how long everyday tasks take. Or put a friend or family member in charge of a timer and practice guessing at how long you have been engaged in different tasks.

- Call your local school district's special-education chairperson for information about rehabilitative games and activities. Find out if a specialist is available to do private tutoring.

- If you have children, observe how they learn best. This can help you to develop your own learning strategies.

- Use board games such as Monopoly, Scrabble, and Clue, and card games like Go Fish!, gin rummy, and poker, which develop planning, sequencing, and judgment skills. The more you practice, the better your skills will become.

- Ask your local software dealer about various programs from The Learning Company that teach thinking skills.

- Set realistic goals for improvement. Your doctor or rehabilitation therapist can help you do this.

- Expect splinter areas of recovery. For example, you may find you are able to read with comprehension before you regain your social skills.

Problems with your ability to reason, plan, and understand can significantly affect your frustration level and your ability to work and maintain social relationships. While recovery from executive function problems can be slow and erratic, it helps to know that there is a valid reason for your sudden deficits. It is also reassuring to know that professional assistance is available to supplement the coping strategies that you develop on your own or learn from others.

16

SPEECH AND LANGUAGE

John, a 45-year-old car salesman from New Hampshire, was a passenger in a car involved in a rear-end collision. When the police arrived and saw that no one was injured, they asked the questions necessary to complete the accident report. Responding to their questions, John was more talkative than usual but, to his amazement, he had great difficulty retrieving the words he needed for his answers.

A few weeks later at the car dealership, John's boss took him to task for his declining sales performance. While they were talking, the boss realized that John's manner of speaking had changed dramatically—that the once-articulate salesman sounded less sophisticated than before and was peppering his speech with nonsense words. John, however, was aware only of a slight word-finding problem.

As months went by, John's language difficulties increased. He consulted his family physician, who referred him to a psychiatrist, believing that stress was the culprit. Meanwhile, John's job performance became so poor that he was laid off, and his overall anxiety about finances and his now-obvious language problem made matters even worse. Eventually, John decided to seek another medical opinion, which led to neurological testing and the discovery that his word-retrieval problem was due to a mild brain injury. John is still unemployed, but he is working with a speech/language therapist at a rehabilitation hospital to try to regain his former verbal skills.

Speech problems, or difficulties using the tongue, lips, palate, and larynx to produce sounds, are a common enough occurrence in everyday life. So are deficits in the ability to use and understand language. However, problems of this kind rarely appear suddenly, as they can following an MTBI—a circumstance that can easily overwhelm you if you must suddenly scramble at home and on the job to compensate for mysteriously absent verbal skills.

WHY SPEECH AND LANGUAGE PROBLEMS CAN OCCUR AFTER AN MTBI

Several areas of the brain help to govern your ability to form words, express yourself, and understand spoken language. Even microscopic nerve-cell damage in one of these areas can disrupt your ability to process the auditory stimuli that precede and accompany verbal communication. Injury to the lower left hemisphere of the frontal lobe can damage Broca's area—one of your speech centers—and hamper articulation (the ability to pronounce speech sounds) and fluency (the ability to combine sounds and words smoothly). If other parts of the frontal lobe bear the brunt of the blow, both your ability to concentrate on what you are saying and your attentiveness to the conversation of others may be affected. In general, you may be less able to use or understand verbal or written communication.

Damage to Wernicke's area, located in the upper left hemisphere of the temporal lobe, can impair your ability to hear and interpret spoken words. You may have trouble understanding language and thus speak nonsense words out of context to the conversation. Language problems can also result if undetectable tearing or stretching of nerve-cell fibers hampers your powers of concentration and your ability to store and retrieve information. In addition, right temporal lobe damage can cause difficulties with nonverbal communication, which involves gestures, body posture, facial expressions, and eye contact.

SPEECH AND LANGUAGE PROBLEMS THAT CAN FOLLOW MTBI

"Before my MTBI, I spoke in a rapid-fire fashion and was fond of embellishing my speech with lots of vivid analogies. Afterward, I spoke slowly, deliberately, and in a noticeably concrete manner. While this tendency has faded over time, I still sometimes use a word or expression incorrectly. I also have an intermittent word-retrieval problem. Interestingly, my son Craig has a learning disability that is characterized by a similar word-finding problem. These days, we communicate beautifully! He says, "Mom, may I have one of the yellow things on the shelf?" and without hesitation, I walk toward the bowl of bananas."

—D.R.S.

"I spent two days trying to come up with the English word for melanzane. *I could see the eggplant and picture it in recipes, but could think of only its*

Italian name. If I continue to picture an object without asking someone or looking it up, the name will eventually come on its own. Stuttering happens most when I'm thinking and can't keep up with the speed of the conversation. I've learned to stay relaxed, slow down my tongue, and let things catch up."
—Elizabeth

The types of communication difficulties related to MTBI can be as different in form and degree as in origin. Whatever your deficit, it is likely to have an impact on every aspect of daily living. To help you better understand your sudden struggles with speech and language, the most commonly encountered problems are described below.

Speech Problems

There are three main types of speech problems that occur after MTBI: verbal apraxia, dysarthria, and dysfluency. *Verbal apraxia* is characterized by the inability to produce purposeful sounds or words on command, even though there are no muscular problems that would interfere with speech. This problem can cause you to sound as if you are stuttering, or as if you are having problems with word-finding.

Dysarthria is often characterized by problems with the muscle movements needed to form, or articulate, words. It can also affect pronunciation of spoken sounds. *Dysfluency,* better known as stuttering, takes the form of hesitant, stammering pronunciation of the beginning sounds of spoken words. Usually there are a number of "false starts," as you repeatedly utter the initial sound or syllable of a word, but the rest of the word fails to follow. Or you may involuntarily draw out single sounds for several seconds as you attempt to summon the rest of the word. Dysfluency after MTBI is most often seen in people who stuttered as children, though it is not known why such an injury can cause stuttering to resurface.

Language Problems

Aphasia is an impairment in the ability to understand or express words or their nonverbal equivalents. There are many different types of aphasia, but most fall into one of three categories: expressive, receptive, and mixed.

Expressive aphasia involves problems with spelling, sentence structure, verbal reasoning, and/or the rate of speech. The most common type of expressive aphasia is known as *Broca's aphasia*. With this type of aphasia, a person is able to understand language but unable to produce speech fluently. Instead, words are spoken in a telegraphic manner, using single words and gestures to convey meaning. For example, a person with Broca's aphasia talking about a plane trip might say, "Plane. . . me. . . . " and spread his or her arms like wings to make the point. Broca's aphasia also involves the inability to repeat or write things that are heard.

Another type of expressive aphasia is *neologism,* a condition marked by grammatical confusions, inappropriate word usage, and the substitution of nonsense words for real words. *Anomia,* a third form of expressive aphasia, renders a person completely unable to name familiar objects, almost as if he or she were suddenly required to converse in a foreign language. A lesser form of this problem is *dysnomia,* which causes you to grope for words that you know but simply can't think of. "It's on the tip of my tongue," and "You know, the whaddayacallit" are statements characteristic of people with word-retrieval problems.

Fluent aphasia is a type of expressive aphasia that results in speech that is properly pronounced, grammatically correct, and effortlessly produced. However, it is often rapid, excessively wordy, and lacking in meaningful content. *Conductive aphasia* is characterized by halting speech with word-finding pauses and concrete rephrasing of words. *Perseverative speech* involves remaining on a topic or the uncontrolled repetition of words, phrases, sentences, or ideas.

Receptive aphasia is a term that denotes problems with reading, interpreting, and comprehending spoken language. Also called *Wernicke's aphasia,* this problem affects the understanding of the meaning of spoken and written words. Your ability to articulate words may be unaffected, but even though you may be able to recognize the conversation of others, you may be unable to comprehend it, almost as if they were speaking a foreign language. Or you may be able to comprehend, but find yourself struggling to process one aspect of what is being said and missing much of the subsequent conversation. You may also engage in a great deal of meaningless verbalization.

Paraphasia is a type of receptive aphasia characterized by the substition of parts of words or syllables for real words. *Alexia,* another form of receptive aphasia, is the inability to understand written language. *Dyslexia* involves difficulties with reading (more about this in Chapter 17). *Mixed aphasia* is a problem with both the comprehension and expression of language.

DIAGNOSING SPEECH AND LANGUAGE PROBLEMS

Successful verbal communication requires that several neurological events occur simultaneously. A malfunction in any facet of the intake or transmission of nerve impulses can have a far-reaching effect. Because the result can be frightening, frustrating, and a significant handicap to job performance and everyday functioning, it is wise to investigate the cause of any speech or language deficits that follow your MTBI.

Your primary health-care provider may recommend an MRI or CT scan, though these tests usually yield negative results in MTBI cases. (See Chapter 2 for a detailed discussion of these procedures.) You may wish to ask about an EEG, which can be significant if it shows a slowing of brain waves in the temporal lobe. You will probably be given a referral to a neurologist, and you should ask for a neuropsychological assessment as well. This evaluation should be able to pinpoint the underlying source of speech or language difficulties, and provide a starting point for the formulation of a rehabilitation program.

TREATING MTBI-RELATED SPEECH AND LANGUAGE PROBLEMS

Articulation and stuttering problems that are aftereffects of MTBI often disappear on their own within three months. Language deficits may fade more slowly and require additional help. What follows is a look at conventional and alternative approaches to resolving communication problems that are slow to correct themselves.

Conventional Approaches

If your neurologist feels that intervention is indicated because of your lifestyle or the degree of your speech or language impairment, therapy with a speech/language pathologist is likely to be the first step. This type of therapy helps you learn to work around your deficits, stimulate or retrain your brain's speech centers, and monitor the redevelopment of your verbal skills, as needed. EMG biofeedback can also be very effective for improving speech; it teaches you to identify and recognize individual muscle movements in and around your mouth.

Psychotherapy may be suggested to help you cope with the frustration of feeling misunderstood and being unable to express yourself. Family counseling can also be helpful as a means of promoting patience and understanding, and teaching strategies for assisting the person with MTBI.

Alternative Approaches

There are no established alternative treatments for expressive or receptive language problems. However, acupuncture by a licensed acupuncturist has been shown to improve articulation. Polarity therapy has been known to help stuttering in some cases. This hands-on technique should be applied by a trained polarity therapist. The American Polarity Therapy Association (see the Resources list at the end of the book) should be able to refer you to a practitioner in your area.

PRACTICAL SUGGESTIONS

"I found that by reading aloud for one hour every day, slowly repeating any words I stumbled on, I was finally able to say them correctly without stuttering. I used humor a lot, too. When I stuttered really badly on a word, I would grin and add, 'That's easy for you to say!' or even, 'Just call me Porky.'"

—Julia

At home and work, you can become practiced at analyzing your speech or language problems. Do you seem to struggle the most when you are fatigued or pressed for time? Are your thoughts disorganized, or does your problem seem to be purely physical? Examining all aspects of your struggle to communicate can point the way to helpful coping strategies, such as those that follow:

- To relax yourself and cut down on stuttering caused by stress, try inhaling deeply through your nose and exhaling through your mouth.

- Eliminate distractions to conversation. Your speech will flow more smoothly and you will have an easier time with comprehension if you talk in a quiet place.

- Gain a measure of control over stuttering by reading aloud to yourself, using a tape recorder and headphones. Start slowly and gradually increase your speed so that you learn to recognize—and then avoid—the point at which you start to stutter.

- Ask a friend or family member to give a prearranged signal when you are going off on a tangent or failing to make sense in conversation. A friend can also stand by at social gatherings to supply key words that escape you.

- Be honest about your problem both at work and at home. This will help you avoid embarrassment and promote patience and understanding in people who might otherwise judge you harshly.

- Temper any tendencies toward outspokenness for now, and avoid becoming involved in friendly debates. Doing so will save you a great deal of frustration.

- Try to visualize an elusive word as if it were written on a chalk-board, or try to hear the word in your head. If you still cannot retrieve the word, describe it or substitute another.

- Use a computer to communicate. Helpful software is widely available, including children's language games and programs and the *American Heritage Dictionary*'s word-finding feature.

- Explore drawing, music, dance, journal-writing, and the theater as ways to help redevelop your language skills. Being inventive can help you think of many activities that stretch your ability to express yourself.

- Consider working with educational card and board games geared toward elementary-school children. Contact the special-education department of your local public school system for specific suggestions and other helpful ideas.

- Watch movies with the sound turned off for practice interpreting gestures, expressions, body movements, and other forms of non-verbal communication.

- If your problem is an expressive one, consider learning American Sign Language as a temporary means of restoring your much-needed ability to communicate.

It is difficult to accept sudden deficits in speech or language, and very humbling to have to rely on others to help you communicate appropriately. It often helps to look at your verbal deficits as a transient symptom rather than a permanent disability. By seeking professional assistance and family support, developing strategies that work for you, and being realistic about occasional setbacks, you will pave the way for certain improvement in your speech and language skills.

17

ACADEMIC PERFORMANCE

Joe, a 22-year-old mechanic, was a writer and an amateur musician. At work one day, he was struck on the top of the head by a wrench. The young man's head ached and he complained of dizziness but he was back on the job the next day. A few weeks later, Joe suddenly lost his ability to read music. And though he could write both spontaneous and dictated text in a perfectly normal manner, Joe found copying music or written passages to be strangely difficult. His struggles were compounded by a sense of despair. It took time and a great deal of patience, but Joe's reading and writing skills have shown significant improvement. Five years later, Joe has returned to his beloved music—a hobby he once feared he would have to abandon.

Given the wide range of possible aftereffects of MTBI, you shouldn't be surprised if you find yourself faltering academically following an accident of this type. You may struggle to understand or perform calculations. Or you may encounter reading comprehension problems, spelling difficulties, or a diminished ability to write. Naturally, such conditions have an adverse effect on school or job performance, and are likely to trouble you at home as well.

WHY ACADEMIC PERFORMANCE CAN SUFFER AFTER MTBI

Your brain is an intricate organ that governs the multitude of skills that are part of academic competency. As you would expect, the academic deficits that can surface after MTBI vary, depending on the site and extent of nerve-cell damage within the brain. With reading, writing, spelling, or math problems, the location of injury is believed to be the area between the back of the left parietal lobe and the left occipital lobe (see Chapter 1). Problems with recognition of faces and symbols, social relationships, dancing, and creative expression are believed to originate in the corresponding area of the brain's right hemisphere.

If the temporal lobe is affected by MTBI, some degree of short- or long-term memory loss often occurs. If this happens, you may encounter related problems with word and letter identification, reading comprehension, or remembering and applying the principles of phonics. If the back of the brain received the impact, the occipital lobe may be injured. This part of the brain oversees vision and recognition. Problems with eye movement and eye-hand coordination can result, as can difficulties with perception and with recalling words.

ACADEMIC PERFORMANCE PROBLEMS
THAT CAN FOLLOW MTBI

"I was an avid reader prior to my accident, plowing through some 3,000 words per minute with 90-percent comprehension. Suddenly, I couldn't read simple instructions! Sometimes I could see the letters but had no idea what the words were or what they meant. At other times, I could read and understand, but couldn't recall what I had read just a few minutes before. My math skills were affected, too. I was shocked to find that I—a former cost-accounting instructor at a local college—was unable to perform computations and fathom monetary values. It was four and a half years before I could go to lunch with a friend and calculate my share of the bill!"

—D.R.S.

The brain trauma caused by MTBI has the potential to diminish a number of academic skill areas, and can be linked to certain specific deficits in reading, writing, spelling, and math. The problems of this type that are encountered most often are described below.

Reading Problems

Reading difficulties can stem from several different sources. If your MTBI has interfered with eye movements, you may struggle to focus or have trouble tracking—that is, following the text from one line of print to the next. If your memory has been affected, you are likely to have trouble recognizing letters or words and retaining the information you have just read. Or you may encounter a processing difficulty such as *dyslexia*, which can cause misperception of letters and letter sequences, misidentification of words, and an inability to distinguish text from its background. You may also have problems following visual sequences and doing puzzles.

Alexia, or word blindness, another processing problem, makes you unable to recognize letters or words. As a result, printed words appear as meaningless groups of marks or symbols on the page. *Agnosia alexia* is the complete inability to understand written words, a result of damage to the left occipital lobe.

Writing Problems

Writing problems can be muscle-related, resulting in problems with fine motor movement (the movement of your fingers, hand, or wrist) or coordination. Depending on the location of your MTBI, you may also have trouble coordinating your eyes and hands, which makes copying extremely difficult.

Dysgraphia, another writing disability, results from injury to the parietal lobe that disrupts the transmission of nerve impulses between the hand and brain. As a result, you are unable to perform the motor movements necessary for legible handwriting. If you are suddenly dysgraphic, you may be unable to recall what letters and numbers look like, or how to reproduce them.

Agraphia is a nerve-disconnection problem that interferes with your ability to get your hand to write legibly—or at all, in some cases. Another writing problem is *agitographia,* which is characterized by very rapid writing movements that cause letters, words, or parts of words to be distorted or omitted.

Spelling Problems

Spelling difficulties that follow MTBI can have several causes. If your visual memory has been impaired, for instance, you may find yourself forgetting what certain words—or even certain letters of the alphabet—look like. Auditory memory problems can adversely affect your "sounding-out" skills by interfering with your recall of letter sounds, word sounds, and the rules of phonics. *Alexia agraphia* is a disability marked by an inability to identify and reproduce letters, words, and numbers. This condition completely undermines any attempts at spelling.

Math Problems

You may find that your ability to use and understand numerals, mathematical symbols, musical notes, and other symbols has been diminished as a result of your MTBI. This disorder, called *dyssymbolia,* can cause you to struggle to comprehend prices, sizes, measurements, and other everyday numerical concepts. Another skill impairment, *dyscalculia,* affects your ability to add, subtract, multiply, and divide—both on paper and in your head. Visual memory problems, another common occurrence after MTBI, can diminish your recall of the rules behind fractions, decimals, percentages, and other higher-level math concepts.

DIAGNOSING ACADEMIC PERFORMANCE PROBLEMS

While deficits in reading, writing, spelling, or using numbers are easy to recognize—and, when they appear suddenly, to link with an MTBI—it can nevertheless be difficult to determine the exact source of such problems. Impaired writing skills, for example, can stem either from problems with your hand muscles or from parietal-lobe damage. Mathematical disabilities can originate in the left or the right side of the brain. In addition, your diminished skills may stem from a combination of problems—say, impaired eye-hand coordination combined with visual memory loss—rather than from injury to just one area of the brain.

If your MTBI has left you with academic problems, your physician or other health-care provider should refer you to a neuropsychologist for evaluation. You will be interviewed, examined, and given a battery of tests to assess various cognitive and academic skills and compare them with your previous level of functioning. The results should determine the nature and extent of your problems and point the way toward treating and overcoming your deficits.

TREATING MTBI-RELATED
ACADEMIC PERFORMANCE PROBLEMS

"I could hold a pen, but could not get my hand to make the writing movements I wanted it to make. Yet I could operate my computer with little difficulty. This helped me to record my thoughts and feelings, communicate, and learn to read again. Later, when I could write again, I found that gesturing with my other hand helped me to improve my spelling. I also took a multisensory approach to spelling, tracing words in sand and asking family members to write on my back with their fingertips."

—D.R.S.

Time is a great healer of academic problems caused by MTBI, since most problems improve in the first six months. However, since skills of this nature are often needed on the job—and are always required to perform at-home responsibilities—most people with MTBI are reluctant to simply wait out the recovery process. Happily, help is widely available.

There are special study drills and other therapeutic activities that can help you improve or regain faltering academic abilities. If necessary, you can also be helped to find ways to circumvent deficient skills. A learning-disabilities specialist or other special educator can help you set reasonable goals throughout your recovery, suggest materials and exercises, and work with you to help you attain these goals. Your doctor, local school district, or a nearby rehabilitation hospital should be able to refer you to a specialist trained to work with people with MTBIs. There are many specific treatment techniques that may be used, depending on your particular problems and individual learning style. For instance, if you learn best through tactile input, or feeling things, a program to remediate calculation problems would involve manipulatives, or materials that teach the skill through touch.

Occupational therapy may be recommended, especially if you need to overcome visual or small-muscle impairments or learn new techniques for dispatching troublesome tasks at work. In addition, psychotherapy and family counseling can help you cope with the feelings of frustration and despair that can stem from finding yourself with suddenly diminished academic abilities.

PRACTICAL SUGGESTIONS

"My solution for dealing with the problem of transposing letters and numbers was to spend time entering recipes and gardening notes into the computer. There has been very noticeable improvement, which has stayed, for the most part. I also discovered that my concentration was affected by various musical backgrounds, and that I seemed to concentrate better with Mozart and classical jazz."

—Elizabeth

While you put your doctor's or practitioner's advice to work against faltering academic skills, you can also take steps on your own to make life easier during your recovery period. The tried-and-true suggestions that follow can help you get started.

- Make grocery lists from supermarket circulars and compare the costs of various items. This not only exercises your numerical skills, but allows you to do comparison shopping ahead of time and at your own pace.

- Use a computer to store ideas, lists, schedules, reminders, and notes about just-read material. When your memory fails you, the computer can recall the needed information (and unlike a piece of paper, is unlikely to be mislaid).

- Look into computer hardware and software that can help you compensate for specific deficits. Soundproof from HumanWare Inc., for example, provides a small voice synthesizer and a tracking device that lets you hear what appears on the monitor rather than having to read it. Xerox produces a scanner that copies pages of text onto the screen to be read to you.

- Carry a pocket-sized calculator with you at all times to help with difficult math calculations and money management.

- If making change confuses you, consider paying for most items by check or credit card.

- Consult a remedial reading or math teacher for ideas and materials to help you design strategies to compensate for lagging skills. Also consider employing a tutor. Your local school district should be able to provide the necessary referrals. A reading program such as those offered by Evelyn Wood Reading Dynamics may also be useful (see the Resources section at the end of this book).

- Check toy stores, educational materials stores, and your local public library for electronic games, board games, workbooks, and other materials that can help you exercise the skills that are giving you trouble.

- If reading is a problem, borrow books on tape from your local public library or order them from Books on Tape (see the Resources section at the end of the book).

- Consider investing in a notebook computer or voice-activated tape recorder to offset writing and note-taking problems. Voice-activated computers are also available.

- Try reading instructions, lists, recipes, and other printed material aloud to compensate for visual memory or comprehension problems.

- Put a triangular pencil grip around your writing implements to achieve better control. Or try using a wide-barreled pen or a chunky beginner's pencil.

- Use flash cards designed for preschoolers to help with word or symbol recognition needed for spelling or math. A number 5 card, for example, might show five objects next to the numeral, clearly depicting the concept of "how many?"

- To help with spelling problems, investigate electronic devices such as Franklin's Spelling Ace, which provides the correct spellings for typed-in approximations.

It is distressing to suddenly lose your ability to enjoy a novel, compose a letter, take notes, or do math computations. Problems of this nature that result from MTBI often fade over time; however, it makes little sense to simply wait out the recovery process. Instead, be honest about the skill areas that trouble you, be aggressive about finding the right professional assistance, and concentrate on formulating helpful strategies and shortcuts to offset your disability. Your take-charge efforts will spark more rapid improvement and do wonders for your state of mind as well.

PART FOUR

EMOTIONAL ASPECTS

INTRODUCTION

Twenty-eight-year-old Shari, an operating-room nurse from Andover, Massachusetts, was involved in a crash with an eighteen-wheel truck. Several ambulances arrived at the scene, but Shari felt fine and insisted that she was okay. In fact, one of her friends took her out for breakfast and then drove her home.

At first, the only symptom Shari noticed was severe muscle pain. Later, when she complained of irritability, crying spells, and mood swings, doctors said her emotionality was a reaction to her discomfort. It was not until five or six months later, when Shari began experiencing sensory overload and blackouts, that she was referred to a neurologist. Within minutes, the neurologist diagnosed a mild traumatic brain injury.

In the years that followed, Shari experienced emotional instability and feelings of sadness and grief. For a time, she saw a clinical psychologist at a local rehabilitation hospital. In addition, she joined the hospital's mild traumatic brain injury support group, which helped a great deal. At present, Shari is back at work on a part-time basis. She recently had her third child and is enjoying life, though she is still recovering from her MTBI.

Part Four of this book deals with the emotional and psychological aspects of MTBI. In some ways, the psychological aspect is more complicated than either the physical or mental aspect. First of all, emotional and psychological symptoms can be more difficult to recognize and describe. If you are having headaches, for instance, you will probably know immediately that something is wrong and why the problem is occurring. With emotional and psychological symptoms, this is not always the case. To begin with, you may have trouble recognizing that what you are experiencing—say, frequent bursts of anger—is not an ordinary emotion, but a sign that something is wrong. Then, once you do identify an emotional or psychological symptom, you may find it difficult and/or embarrassing to try to discuss this with your physician.

Further complicating the situation is the fact that many emotional and psychological symptoms can have more than one underlying cause. Sometimes they result directly from injury to the brain; other times they may be a secondary reaction to brain trauma. They can also be a side effect of medications prescribed for MTBI symptoms, or they can represent an exacerbation of a previously existing psychological disorder.

Take the example of depression, which can result from several conditions. It may be caused by injury to the frontal lobe, a part of the brain involved in mood. Or you may be unable to continue working and, as a result, feel depressed. Or, if you have migraines or cluster headaches following an MTBI, your doctor may prescribe a beta-blocker as a preventive, and the beta-blocker may cause depression as a side effect. Finally, if you had occasional mild but manageable depressive episodes prior to your injury, you may find yourself facing major depression afterward. Thus, any one one of four different scenarios—or any combination thereof—can lead to the same result. In addition, some emotional and psychological symptoms can cause and/or be part of others. For example, depression can cause reduced sex drive, which can in turn lead to difficulty in personal relationships.

If you think this sounds confusing, you're right—it can be, but Part Four will provide you with some direction. The most common emotional and psychological effects of MTBI are considered here in four groups: postinjury reactions; mood and behavior problems; the magnification of preexisting psychological disorders; and grieving. However, you should keep in mind that, as described above, it is possible for a single symptom to have more than one cause, and as such to have a place in more than one of the four groups.

With the assistance of health-care practitioners who have experience in treating MTBI, it should be possible to identify the underlying cause of your distress. The good news is that for most of these problems, there are treatments that can help.

18

POSTINJURY
PSYCHOLOGICAL
REACTIONS

Wyoming resident Nancy was involved in a minor auto accident. The impact caused her to bump her head, but based on her appearance and behavior, police at the scene told her she could go home. Weeks later, Nancy resigned from her job, which had suddenly become quite stressful. But at home, things were no better. Nancy, who had always been careful about money, began to lose bills or fail to pay them on time. She was unable to balance her checkbook. She decided to try her hand at cosmetic sales, and bought $3,500 worth of skin- and hair-care products without a single customer. At night, she would wake up from a sound sleep, drenched in perspiration and feeling jittery and upset.

Eventually, Nancy took a new job, but it lasted only two weeks. She couldn't put her finger on the problem, but things in her life just didn't feel right. At yet another job a few months later, Nancy's work pace was pitifully slow. She was afraid to answer the phone, unable to make decisions, and found herself getting up in the middle of the night to tackle unfinished work. Convinced that she was going crazy, Nancy sought professional help, only to discover that she was having a psychological reaction to an MTBI.

Life experiences, whether normal or out of the ordinary, create physical and psychological stimulation that summon responses from both body and mind. Upon failing a test, you might flush with embarrassment and feel defensive or guilty. Faced with losing a job or relationship, you may tremble and sweat and feel awash in self-reproach. These reactions show that circumstances have pushed you beyond your tolerance level and that your defenses have been activated. It should not surprise you to learn that psychological reactions can easily be triggered by the physical and emotional upheaval of an MTBI.

WHY POSTINJURY PSYCHOLOGICAL REACTIONS OCCUR

Much as your immune system kicks in in response to a deep cut or an infection, the circumstances and aftermath of brain trauma ignite psychological responses. Physical and emotional pain that exceed your personal threshold can make you feel nauseated or numb, or even make you faint. Such physical reactions are often part of psychological upheaval.

Psychological responses also commonly involve emotional, cognitive, or behavioral elements. Emotional elements may include denial, avoidance, anxiety, emotional numbness, and/or feelings of grief or guilt. Cognitive reactions may take the form of rationalizing, blaming, and/or being judgmental. Behavioral elements may include aggressiveness, expressions of anger, withdrawal, diminished abilities, lack of control, and overwhelming sadness. In many cases, behavioral responses develop into physical symptoms such as headaches, ulcers, chest pain, sleep problems, or suppression of the immune system.

Extraordinary life experiences, including such unexpected and traumatic occurrences as fire, assault, or automobile accidents, often lead to posttraumatic stress. The same is true of MTBI. This can be experienced immediately, as acute stress, or as a delayed response months or even years later.

WHAT POSTINJURY PSYCHOLOGICAL REACTIONS ARE LIKE

MTBI is often experienced as a personal disaster. You may have feelings of defeat, frustration, and inadequacy. In addition, you may suffer anxiety over your sudden lack of control over things and the sense that you have failed yourself and your family.

When your mind and body are out of harmony or balance, a distress signal is sent to indicate danger to you. This may take the form of pain. To avoid feeling this pain, your mind's or body's reaction is to shut down through an initial reaction of numbness. Following this shut-down phase is another set of responses called the "fight-or-flight" mode. At this point, some people choose the "fight" option—that is, they take the offensive as a way of dealing with MTBI aftereffects, displaying such responses as verbal or physical aggression, angry outbursts, and blaming others. Others choose "flight"; their psychological response is to withdraw, flee, or psychologically defend themselves against the realization of sudden personal changes. This withdrawal can take different forms, including physical withdrawal (such as literally running away from an accident scene), denial (refusing to believe the injury happened), rationalization (coming up with an explanation of its cause), or guilt (blaming oneself).

In most situations, psychological responses are not displayed in separate parts, but as a mixture of reactions. For instance, if you were injured in an automobile accident, it might be emotionally easier for you to express feelings of anger at the other driver (aggressiveness) and to insist that the crash was his fault (rationalizing and blaming) than it would be either to acknowledge that you might be to blame or to focus your thoughts on the disabilities you now face. This is especially true if such an acknowledgment might be painful—say, if alcohol or drugs were involved, or if a loved one was injured while you were behind the wheel, or if you must deal with a permanent physical disability of some kind.

Another possible response to MTBI is posttraumatic stress disorder (PTSD). With this syndrome, you find yourself involuntarily reliving the traumatic experience in your mind. You may also experience nightmares, feelings of overwhelming helplessness and anxiety, nervous alertness, distractibility, and depression. If you also have amnesia, instead of experiencing intrusive memories and flashbacks you may experience emotional or bodily sensations evoked by sounds, colors, temperatures, or other stimuli that are in some way related to the accident. For instance, cracking ice might be upsetting because it mimics the sound of breaking glass. The reactions to PTSD may be heightened if the disaster was life-threatening and caused you to feel overwhelmingly vulnerable.

Whatever direction psychological reactions take, feelings of guilt and shame over the inability to live life as before are common. These emotions can leave you isolated, reproachful, and filled with self-doubt. They can be compounded by a prior history of coping problems, which makes psychological distress more likely, or by the malaise that accompanies chronic fatigue.

DIAGNOSING POSTINJURY PSYCHOLOGICAL REACTIONS

Not all psychological reactions are severe or long-lasting enough to require professional intervention. But because brain trauma, depression, and denial can cloud your judgment, and because the range of potential emotional and psychological symptoms that can occur in the aftermath of an MTBI is so broad, you may not be the best person to assess your own situation.

For the most accurate and objective diagnosis, you should consult a mental health professional who has training and experience in both trauma and brain injury. Symptoms such as aggression, depression, and suicidal thinking can be the result of organic brain injury (more about this in Chapter 19), a postinjury psychological response, and/or posttraumatic stress disorder. In order to get proper treatment, it is extremely important to know what is behind your symptoms.

TREATING POSTINJURY PSYCHOLOGICAL REACTIONS

As mentioned above, postinjury psychological reactions do not necessarily require treatment. Professional help is certainly indicated if reactions become severe and/or prolonged enough to interfere with daily living. But even if your postinjury reactions are not that severe, you may find treatment to be very beneficial for your recovery and for your life in general.

Because these problems are often multifaceted, treatment through a team approach is usually recommended. Depending on your circumstances, your neurologist may refer you to a neuropsychologist, a psychiatrist, a psychologist, and/or a psychopharmacologist. You may also receive assistance from a clinical social worker, rehabilitation counselor, and, if needed, a case manager. Patient and family counseling and training can be very effective.

Conventional Approaches

Psychotherapy can be extremely valuable for coming to an understanding of, and working through, psychological reactions to injury. Behavioral medicine—specifically, hypnotherapy and trauma therapy—may be used. EEG biofeedback is helpful for dealing with depression and the symptoms of PTSD. Cognitive-behavioral therapy can help you to modify your thought patterns, change problem behavior, and deal with psychological trauma. (See Chapter 3 for a complete discussion of these therapeutic approaches.)

These types of therapy should be conducted by a licensed psychologist or psychiatrist. For the therapy to be effective, it is crucial to find an appropriate medical or mental health care provider. This person should be compassionate, caring, well trained, and experienced with your type of problem. Finding the right person may be difficult, especially in less populated areas where the supply of well-trained people may be limited. However, it is vital for your outcome to find someone who believes you can get better and is willing to work with you.

In addition to one-on-one therapy, support groups work well for brain-injured people. There are four basic types of support groups. The first, a self-help group led by a trained facilitator, can educate a person with MTBI and his or her family as to who the MTBI person has become. The second type of support group is informational in nature, and invites outside speakers and others to make presentations to the group on relevant topics. A third, more therapeutic, type of support group provides a trained counselor who helps members deal with their emotions and progress through the various stages of grieving and healing. The fourth type, more often used in cases of severe and moderate head injury, serves as a training group for family members involved in home health care. A local rehabilitation center or the Brain Injury Association (see the Resources section beginning on page 281) should be able to furnish information about support groups in your area.

Your doctor may recommend medication to help you cope with your postinjury psychological reactions. Depending on your symptoms, there are a number of medications, such as antidepressants, anticonvulsants, mood stabilizers, and beta-blockers, that can help. The exact medication or combination of medications appropriate for your needs will depend on the nature and cause of your problem, as well as on your individual biochemical makeup. To ensure that you obtain proper care, medication, and dosages, it is wise to see a psychopharmacologist who specializes in MTBI.

Alternative Approaches

Polarity therapy, which helps to bring the mind and body into better harmony, can help you deal with psychological reactions to your MTBI. This type of therapy should be provided by a trained practitioner. The American Polarity Therapy Association (see the Resources section at the end of the book) should be able to provide a referral to a polarity therapist in your area.

There are herbal and homeopathic preparations that can be beneficial for some postinjury psychological reactions. However, to determine what is right for you, it is best to consult with a qualified herbalist or homepathic practitioner who specializes in MTBI and PTSD. At first, treating some postinjury psychological symptoms may seem easy; you know if you are feeling sad, anxious, or whatever. But as with headaches, the underlying causes can vary widely, so remedies of any kind should be used with care. If you are depressed, for example, taking the wrong product could cause a more severe depression. If your physician is unable to help you or to refer you to an appropriate practitioner, the Herb Research Foundation or the National Center for Homeopathy (see the Resources section at the end of this book) should be able to help.

Other types of alternative treatments that may help your symptoms include massage therapy, acupressure, aromatherapy, and flower essence therapy. Beyond helping your muscles to relax, massage therapy may stimulate the blood flow to the brain, aiding in the healing process. Acupressure, using finger pressure on the body, hands, feet, or ears, can release blocks in the flow of *chi,* or vital energy. There are books, such as Diane Stein's *The Natural Remedy Book for Women* (Crossing Press, 1992), that can guide you in this practice, although ideally you should consult with a licensed acupuncturist before trying to treat yourself.

Aromatherapy, the use of aromatic essential oils distilled from plants, can be used to help calm and relax you or to boost your energy levels. For example, clary sage is often used for its calming effects, ylang-ylang for relaxation, and cypress for increased energy. Roberta Wilson's *Aromatherapy for Vibrant Health and Beauty* (Avery Publishing Group, 1995) provides specific, easy-to-follow instructions for using this art to treat both physical and emotional conditions.

Unlike essential oils, flower essences do not employ scent. They are closer in nature to homeopathic remedies—highly diluted preparations that contain the imprint of plant energy. Flower-essence therapists believe that the life force of the various flowers can affect both body and mind. Edward Bach, an English homeopath and physician, is the most noted theorist and practitioner of flower-essence therapy. To find out which remedies might best help your symptoms, consult a guide such as *Bach Flower Essences for the Family* (Wigmore, 1993)—or, if possible in your area, consult with a flower-essence therapist who is knowledgeable about MTBI.

PRACTICAL SUGGESTIONS

"Pets tend to reteach us uncomplainingly how to touch when you scratch their ears, 'shake hands,' or pet them. I used my cats as my first therapists— they would move out of arm's reach to get me to realize that I had done the petting too roughly."

—Lianne

There is a satisfying sense of control inherent in finding ways to speed your recovery from any MTBI symptom. The suggestions below may help you cope with the psychological aftermath of your injury:

• View informative videos. The Brain Injury Association offers a helpful one about MTBI and postconcussive syndrome. Another video, which debuted as an ABC Sunday Night Movie, is called *A Stranger in the Family.* The Brain Injury Association can help you secure a copy of this video as well.

• Look into interactive communication networks for computers. There are bulletin boards, chat rooms, and forums through such services as Prodigy, America Online (AOL), Microsoft Network (MSN), and CompuServe where a wide range of people with similar problems can find support.

• Pursue a sport or hobby that brings a feeling of accomplishment or comfort. Consider unstructured activities such as gardening or painting that encourage expression and emphasize your personal strengths.

• If you don't already have one, consider getting a pet. Research has shown that pet owners recover faster than those without animal companions. Any type of pet is suitable, provided you can care for it properly. The type you choose should depend on your capabilities and housing situation.

• Avoid activities that require organizational skills and memory, or whatever skill you are having trouble with. Cooking, for instance, is likely to highlight shortcomings in thinking skills and can be extremely frustrating.

• When you feel anxiety or frustration mounting, nip it in the bud by taking a bath, going for a walk, doing yoga, dancing, singing, counting to ten, or using relaxation techniques like deep breathing.

• Avoid the use of alcohol or cigarettes to calm yourself. These substances might seem to help in the short term, but they can cause further injury to your body and make many MTBI symptoms worse.

• Do not attempt to medicate yourself with over-the-counter preparations. Overuse or improper dosages may cause further complications.

• Consider spiritual counseling and/or a church-, temple-, or mosque-based support group. Most houses of worship offer or can refer you to some kind of community support group.

You will surely discover additional ways of coping, adjusting, and regaining your sense of purpose and self. As you recover from your MTBI, an understanding mental health specialist can be a great source of strength. It is vital to keep searching until you find such a professional. Remember: The road you are on is not an easy one, but you need never travel it alone.

19

MOODS AND BEHAVIOR

Kevin, a 40-year-old Massachusetts man, sustained several concussions in his youth due to football injuries. He recalls only one that seemed to affect him—he was knocked unconscious during a game and diagnosed in the emergency room as having suffered a mild concussion. He was discharged and taken back to the game, but on the school-bus ride home, other students noticed a change in Kevin's behavior. Normally soft-spoken and passive, the boy began swearing a lot and acting rowdy and confrontational. In the locker room the next day, he put his fist through a safety-glass door in an unexplained surge of anger. At the time, no one related Kevin's uncharacteristic behavior to his brain injury. The aggressiveness abated on its own, and he did not display this type of outburst again during his youth.

As an adult, Kevin struck his head again after stumbling over one of his child's toys. The injury seemed minor, but in the days that followed, the old rage returned. At work, Kevin started a fistfight with a man who was vying with him for a parking space. Another time, he flung a cup of coffee across the room when his secretary didn't pour it correctly. At home, he was verbally abusive to his loved ones. Once, he put his fist through the wallboard during an argument.

Eventually, Kevin's uncontrollable anger cost him his job, his girlfriend, and his relationship with his parents. When he sought help, he was diagnosed as having an MTBI and told that his aggression was a result of repeated blows to the head. Since then, Kevin has received medical treatment and psychotherapy. This, along with his participation in a brain-injury support group, has been very effective. Kevin is now working again, has begun a new romantic relationship, and has repaired the ties to his family.

From the time we are children, we are taught that behavior defines a person, and that it is imperative to exercise control over our actions and reactions. If you lose this restraint, suddenly and without apparent cause, it can be terrifying both to you and to your loved ones. It has been shown that mood and behavior changes of this type can have a physical basis—that brain trauma can affect your moods and undermine your ability to check impulses and contain anger. However, you can reestablish self-control and avoid the long-term consequences of inappropriate behavior by understanding why this can occur and by educating yourself about corrective measures.

WHY MOOD AND BEHAVIOR CHANGES CAN OCCUR AFTER MTBI

The brain's frontal lobe helps to govern personality. As a result, an MTBI that causes damage to this area can significantly affect your moods and behavior. The frontal lobe also serves as a braking mechanism; it helps to make you aware when anger is building and allows you to exercise control over your responses. Trauma to the frontal lobe can therefore cause a malfunction in your ability to inhibit aggression.

As described in Chapter 12, an MTBI that causes damage to the temporal lobe sometimes leads to seizures, or irregular discharges of nerve-cell activity. Marked behavior changes—specifically, increased hostility and lack of control over angry outbursts—can be manifestations of temporal-lobe seizure disorder.

MOOD AND BEHAVIOR CHANGES THAT CAN FOLLOW MTBI

"Before my auto accident, I was a calm, patient person who could cope with stress and handle many situations at once. One year after my accident, there was an incident that made me think I was going crazy. I was in a conversation with my teenaged daughter and I suddenly flew into a rage. Shrieking, 'I can't take this anymore!,' I threw papers and my pocketbook ten feet into the air. Then I turned and kicked the back door with such force that I almost broke it."

—Debbie

Over the years, you have developed a sense of appropriateness regarding such emotional displays as tears, anger, or yelling. This learned ability to react in a manner befitting the circumstances is critical to social acceptance as well as to the building of relationships. A frontal- or temporal-lobe injury can interfere with this ability and trigger marked behavior changes. The following are some of the most common problems people with MTBI experience:

- *Intolerance.* After an MTBI, you may find yourself unable to deal with even minor changes in your environment or daily routine without experiencing frustration and, possibly, reacting with unreasonable, almost childish anger.

- *Apathy.* This symptom, which is characterized by extreme indifference and little or no outward emotion, often exists as a function of depression, but it can also be associated with large bilateral frontal-lobe lesions.

- *Misperception of time or events.* MTBI can affect your grasp of time concepts as well as your ability to focus on and assimilate the goings-on around you. Either of these conditions can ignite fear and frustration, which commonly manifest themselves as impatience, extreme irritability, and seemingly self-centered behavior.

- *Difficulty sustaining relationships.* Close personal interactions involve some degree of patience and give-and-take. However, the demanding, clingy, or hostile behavior wrought by your MTBI can quickly erode the fabric of relations with friends and family.

If you undergo a measurable personality change after MTBI, you may be diagnosed with *organic personality change*. This disorder is often characterized by emotional lability (sudden, intense shifts of emotion), impulsivity, suspiciousness, quickness to anger, and frequent verbal outbursts. In other cases, it may manifest itself as listlessness, inattentiveness, and extreme self-involvement. A heightened sensitivity to sound, medications, and alcohol is very common among those affected by this syndrome. Other possible symptoms include excessive talkativeness, immature or otherwise inappropriate social behavior, physical aggression, impatience, poor judgment, eating and drinking problems, distractibility, uncontrollable crying, irritability, excessive dependency, uncontrollable rage, unrealistic optimism, denial of problems, indifference, and violent outbursts.

DIAGNOSING MOOD AND BEHAVIOR CHANGES

It can be difficult to determine whether behavior changes that follow an MTBI are caused by brain trauma, postinjury psychological reactions, or a heightening of preexisting psychiatric problems. For instance, if you are marginally able to cope with feelings of anger before suffering an MTBI, an insult to the brain might further limit your ability to control feelings and behavior, leaving you unable to deal with even small changes in bodily sensations or your environment. Often, the inability to cope is manifested as extreme frustration, anger, and impatience, which can be seen as self-centeredness. In such a case, it is not the symptom itself—the anger—that is a direct result of the injury. Rather, the insult to the brain has limited your ability to control the expression of anger.

As mentioned in the previous section, it can also be difficult to distinguish between the apathy that accompanies organic personality syndrome and disorder, and that which characterizes depression. (More about depression in Chapter 20.) As a further complication, behavioral symptoms and other injury aftereffects, such as attention, concentration, and reasoning deficits, can mimic each other. For example, impulse buying may look like impulsivity, but it may also come about because the selection of appropriate merchandise has suddenly become an ordeal. Similarly, what looks like paranoia may result directly from brain injury, or it may be an individual's response, say, to having the family relieve him or her of bill-paying responsibilities.

Neuropsychological testing is the best means of evaluating the behavioral component of an MTBI, because this battery of tests can distinguish between preexisting personality traits and postinjury reactions in the assessment of symptoms. This type of testing enables the specialist to tailor treatment to the patient, pinpointing the need for speech and language therapy, psychotherapy, or consultation with an audiologist or ophthalmologist. Moreover, neuropsychological testing determines whether rehabilitation (working to restore previous levels of functioning) or compensation (learning ways to live with your deficits) is the appropriate goal.

A test may also be done to rule out malingering (faking illness or injury to achieve some type of gain). This can be very valuable because you may find people questioning whether your postconcussive symptoms are real—especially where legal and insurance-related processes are involved. Many people with MTBI have found themselves suspected of insurance fraud, for example. The test for malingering provides additional information that can help to demonstrate to insurers, employers, or attorneys that your symptoms are real.

TREATING MTBI-RELATED
MOOD AND BEHAVIOR PROBLEMS

"The emotional instability brought on by my MTBI left me feeling out of control. Whereas I rarely cried prior to my accident, I now found myself weeping and becoming extremely irritable for no apparent reason. Concerned about the possibility of depression, I called a psychotherapist who had known me for years and who was also trained in neurology. He urged me to relate my symptoms to my neurologist, who in turn determined that my problems were being

caused by imperceptible seizure activity in my brain. He prescribed a beta-blocker, and within twenty-four hours, all my mood and behavioral symptoms disappeared."

—D.R.S.

Behavioral symptoms that follow MTBI—specifically, mood swings, short-temperedness, and lack of behavioral control—are likely to decrease over time unless a complicating factor such as a seizure condition, posttraumatic stress disorder, or a preexisting psychological disorder is present. In the meantime, there are steps you can take to help control your symptoms and hasten the recovery process.

Conventional Approaches

The first step in treating mood and behavioral problems is to find a behavioral neurologist. This area of neurology specializes in organic personality change. If such a specialist is not available where you live, seek out a psychopharmacologist who has experience treating people with MTBI. This practitioner may suggest various medications, such as anticonvulsants and beta-blockers. Anticonvulsant medications may be used to suppress temporal-lobe seizure activity that can interfere with your regulation of behavior. Beta-blockers can be similarly effective, and are also useful for helping to control your emotions.

Psychotherapy may be recommended to help you learn to manage frustration and make lifestyle modifications to ward off negative behavior. For instance, you may have to restrict your activities and keep socializing to a minimum until you regain emotional and behavioral control. Role-playing and psychodrama are psychological techniques that can help you learn to control outbursts and inappropriate responses. Behavioral medicine and health psychology—in particular, biofeedback and behavior-modification techniques—can be very effective at teaching relaxation.

Alternative Approaches

Polarity therapy can help you to regain a sense of emotional balance. This therapeutic-touch technique should be performed by a trained polarity therapist. The American Polarity Therapy Association (see the Resources section at the end of the book) should be able to provide a referral to a polarity therapist in your area.

There are also over-the-counter herbal and homeopathic remedies that promote relaxation and even-temperedness. You should exercise caution with such products, however, because they are designed for use by the general public, not for controlling mood or behavior problems that follow MTBI. If you wish to try alternative remedies, it is best to consult with a qualified herbalist or homeopathic practitioner, preferably one who has knowledge of organic personality syndrome and MTBI. With this training, the practitioner can tailor a prescription to your unique symptoms and situation. The Herb Research Foundation and/or the National Center for Homeopathy (see the Resources section at the end of the book) may be able to help you locate an appropriate practitioner in your area.

PRACTICAL SUGGESTIONS

"Physical exercise has been instrumental in helping me cope with psychological pain. Not long after my accident, for instance, I was told of the death of a patient I had seen that last day on the job. In turmoil, I walked over two miles until I was able to come to grips with my powerful reaction."

—*D.R.S.*

While professional treatment is critical to your recovery from any MTBI symptom, there is also much you can do on your own to regain a sense of control over your moods and behavior. The following suggestions may be helpful:

- Inform your friends, family, and coworkers about your difficulties with behavior control. Explain to them that any inappropriate behavior you display is temporarily beyond your control and is not to be taken personally. Enlist their support and efforts to shield you from situations that tend to trigger inappropriate responses.

- Ask someone you trust to let you know with a prearranged hand signal, facial expression, or special word when they see you beginning to act out.

- Suggest to coworkers and those close to you that they leave the room rather than confront you when you behave objectionably. Discussion can follow later, when you are calmer.

- Apologize for inappropriate responses. While your behavior is not your fault, it is important to acknowledge that you have been irritable, abusive, or insulting.

- Control verbal outbursts by stopping, breathing deeply, and thinking before you speak. A behavioral therapist can help you learn to do this.

- Avoid people and places that annoy you until you learn methods of controlling your behavior. Understand that normally negative re-actions will be greatly intensified by your MTBI.

- Ask family members and friends to help you respond appropriate-ly by alerting you when a trigger topic must be introduced. For example, "Mary, I know this will be upsetting, but I need to talk about something."

- Remember the effect that inappropriate outbursts have on your fam-ily and friends. They, too, are suffering as a result of your injury.

Injury to the brain frequently produces changes in how people feel and react. However, this symptom is often overlooked. Many people assume that behavioral and mood changes such as excessive anger must be related to a postinjury psychological reaction rather than to the brain injury itself. This can result in crucial delays in obtaining appropriate treatment.

If you, your friends, or members of your family have any ques-tion about mood and behavior changes that occur after an accident or brain injury, obtain a second opinion from a behavioral neurolo-gist or psycholopharmacologist with expertise in MTBI. There is help available.

20

PSYCHIATRIC DISORDERS

Carol, a 24-year-old Mississippi woman, had a history of clinical depression. Her problems had necessitated several hospitalizations over the years, but she had made significant progress. Then, on the way home from a routine appointment with her psychiatrist, Carol was involved in a minor car accident. X-rays were taken at the emergency room, but Carol's injuries were slight and she was sent home.

Days later, severe headaches, memory loss, and uncharacteristic irritability compelled her to see her family physician. Carol also found herself dwelling on thoughts of suicide, but chose not to mention this to either her doctor or her psychiatrist. Based on the symptoms she did discuss, Carol's physician diagnosed a mild traumatic brain injury, and suggested that the young woman consult a neurologist. Before she could do so, however, Carol tried to kill herself, and was subsequently hospitalized at a local psychiatric facility.

The aftereffects of MTBI are pervasive, influencing not only your physical health but your emotional well-being. The connection between brain trauma and the emotions is extremely complex. As we have seen, emotional reactions can result either directly or indirectly from brain injury. This is not the case with psychiatric disorders. Brain injury does not *cause* psychiatric disorders as such, but it can magnify a preexisting problem to the point that your ability to function may be jeopardized. To further complicate matters, symptoms of psychiatric disorders can sometimes mimic those of postconcussive syndrome, making the true nature of the problem difficult to determine.

WHY PSYCHIATRIC PROBLEMS CAN OCCUR AFTER MTBI

To better understand psychiatric disorders, you need to know how they differ from postinjury psychological reactions and organic personality change. In postinjury psychological reactions, your moods and behavior are a response to outside influencing factors. With organic personality change, your moods and behavior are the result of injury to the brain. In contrast, psychiatric disorders are due to heredity, developmental factors, biochemical imbalance, and/or other factors not yet identified.

Some people, like Carol, have had psychiatric symptoms under control through medication and psychotherapy prior to MTBI. In other cases, symptoms of a specific disorder in an individual's family's history may not become apparent until after his or her MTBI. In either situation, psychiatric symptoms are often heightened by MTBI, and can become severe if there is injury to the brain area that controls moods and psychological reactions. Carol, for instance, had been diagnosed with clinical depression resulting from a chemical imbalance. Her accident caused her depression to worsen to the point that she attempted suicide. The most commonly seen psychiatric disorders that may be worsened by MTBI are described below.

Anxiety Disorders

The anxiety disorders include both generalized (chronic) and acute anxiety (panic attacks) and phobias. As discussed in Chapter 18, anxiety is a common reaction in the immediate aftermath of an MTBI, but it can also become a chronic problem that lasts beyond the reaction phase, particularly if you suffered from any degree of anxiety disorder prior to your injury. Phobic disorders are experienced as great anxiety and irrational fear triggered by specific objects or situations. Common examples include *agoraphobia* (fear of open spaces), *claustrophobia* (fear of closed spaces), and *acrophobia* (fear of heights), but virtually anything can be the object of a phobia.

Mood Disorders

Mood disorders are characterized by extreme changes and variations in moods, from depression (profound sadness) to mania (utter elation). Depression is by far the most prevalent psychiatric disorder among people with MTBI. In fact, depression occurs fairly frequently among persons with virtually any type of chronic health problem, and it can lead to a kind of vicious cycle in which depression aggravates your disabilities, which leads to even deeper depression, and so on.

As described in Chapter 18, a temporary depressive reaction is a common occurrence among people in the immediate aftermath of MTBI, as they adjust to the impact that the injury has had on their lives. Clinical depression is longer lasting and more severe than this, and has physical as well as psychological components. Symptoms of clinical depression can include disruptions in your sleep/wake cycle; changes in appetite, with resulting weight loss (or, in some cases, weight gain); pervasive apathy and fatigue; a near-total loss of motivation; loss of sexual interest; an inability to experience pleasure, even from previously enjoyable activities; and thoughts of suicide. Fatigue related to depression is different from fatigue that is a direct result of MTBI, which is described in Chapter 4. With depression-related fatigue, you wake up exhausted and remain exhausted throughout the day. In contrast, with MTBI fatigue, you wake up alert and become fatigued as the day progresses due to cognitive overload and/or physical activity.

Another form of clinical depression can be caused by long-term pain resulting from a traumatic event such as an auto accident. In this situation, it is believed that the signal of and/or a biochemical reaction to ongoing pain triggers depression. If depression is accompanied by persistent bodily pain—such as constant headache, neck, and/or facial pain—for which no physical or psychological cause can be found, you may be diagnosed with clinical depression caused by chronic pain syndrome.

Manic-depressive disorder (known to professionals as mixed-type mood disorder or bipolar depression) involves extreme changes in moods, from deep depression to unrealistic elation and/or hyperactivity and back again. The symptoms of this disorder are sometimes confused with the emotional mood swings that can follow brain injury (see Chapter 19) or severe personal trauma (see Chapter 18).

Sleep Disorders

Most sleep disorders are inherited. Others are related to biochemistry and age. Symptoms of sleep disorders include insomnia and sleep/ wake cycle disturbances as well as other problems related to sleep. If you suffered from such problems before your injury, they may become worse afterward; if you never suffered from sleep disturbances before, it is possible that you may begin to. Many aspects of the aftermath of MTBI can interfere with sleep, including chronic pain, anxiety, depression, circadian-rhythm disturbances, nightmares, sensitivity to noise, and certain medications. In turn, sleep disorders can cause and/or aggravate the extreme fatigue and other problems experienced by people with MTBI.

Substance Abuse

This disorder includes all aspects of drug and alcohol abuse and dependency. If you had a drinking problem before your MTBI, your alcohol abuse is likely to escalate afterward. Drinking and drug use, in turn, contribute to the likelihood that you will suffer an MTBI. A recent survey by the Brain Injury Association showed that the majority of brain injuries are caused by accidents related to drunken driving. In addition, the survey showed that alcohol figures prominently in the high unemployment rate of people with MTBI. In general, the consequences of MTBI can directly affect your ability to cope with chronic social and emotional problems.

Obsessive-Compulsive Disorder

This disorder causes you to feel an uncontrollable need to perform a particular activity over and over again. Some of the compulsive activities most commonly seen include eating, drinking, shopping, gambling, hand-washing, and collecting or checking on things. If you have obsessive-compulsive disorder (OCD), your symptoms are likely to become worse after an MTBI.

Sometimes the coping mechanisms people with MTBI use in response to attention and short-term memory problems can be confused with symptoms of OCD—for instance, keeping things in strict order so that you can find or remember them. This can make a correct diagnosis difficult.

Personality Disorders

A personality disorder is an enduring pattern of exaggeration of an ordinary personality trait, such as a tendency to be self-centered or withdrawn. These exaggerations are considered disorders because they lead to behaviors that interfere with daily living and the maintenance of normal relationships.

In most situations, personality disorders are a result of developmental factors. Often, however, similar behaviors can be explained by brain injury, as seen in interictal behavior (see Chapter 12) or organic personality disorder (see Chapter 19). Types of personality disorders include the following:

- Antisocial (having disregard for others and their rights.)

- Avoidant (withdrawing from social interaction).

- Borderline (impulsive and intrusive).

- Compulsive (having perfectionistic traits).

- Dependent (emotionally needy).

- Histrionic (excessively emotional and attention-seeking).

- Narcissistic (emotionally aloof and lacking remorse).

- Paranoid (overly suspicious).

- Passive-aggressive (behaving placidly, then becoming hostile).

- Schizoid (socially detached).

- Schizotypal (having acute problems with social relationships).

Persons with personality disorders often do not think there is anything wrong with them, and feel their behavior is normal. Friends, family members, and coworkers are more likely to notice the existence of a problem and encourage the individual to seek treatment. In most cases, when personality disorders seem to appear after MTBI, the problem was actually present before the injury in a minor or mild form, and it emerged in response to the stress of the injury and its aftermath.

Psychotic Disorders

These psychiatric disorders are characterized by a split with reality. Symptoms can include delusions, hallucinations, judgment problems, and complete emotional withdrawal, as well as an inability to think clearly or to perceive reality. Probably the best known of the psychotic disorders is *schizophrenia*, which is typified by the symptoms listed above as well as by inappropriate (or absent) emotion and marked memory problems. Most cases of psychotic disorders that appear after MTBI are due to a worsening of previously mild and manageable symptoms, rather than the development of an entirely new illness.

Dissociative Disorders

Dissociative disorders are complex, poorly understood psychiatric disorders in which a person loses conscious awareness of memories, ideas, and feelings—in some cases, even his or her identity—and becomes unable to recall these things. Types of dissociative disorders include *multiple personality disorder* and *psychogenic amnesia*, or memory loss that is a psychological response to emotional stress. With this type of amnesia, the greatest memory loss affects events that were sources of emotional anguish, rather than physical trauma. Like many psychiatric disorders, dissociative disorders most often are not a direct result of brain injury, but can be made worse by it.

Somatoform Disorders

The term *somatoform disorder* refers to the presence of physical complaints for which no physical explanation can be found. Sometimes there are observable symptoms such as vomiting, bloating, or back pain. Other characteristics of somatoform disorder can include imagined defects in appearance; an alteration in physical function suggestive of illness, such as dizziness, headaches, vague chronic pain, or vision problems; and preoccupation with sickness and injury. Like dissociative disorders, somatoform disorders can be exacerbated by MTBI.

Factitious Disorder and Malingering

These two disorders have many features in common. *Factitious disorder* involves intentionally faking some type of illness by inflicting injury on yourself or by pretending to have symptoms that suggest illness, even though you do not stand to gain anything (except, perhaps, a doctor's attention) by doing so. *Malingering* also involves falsifying illness or injury, but with the aim of achieving some sort of benefit, such as being able to avoid work, military duty, or criminal prosecution, or to gain financial compensation. Both of these disorders can become worse following an MTBI.

Disorders of Infancy, Childhood, or Adolescence

These disorders include problems stemming from mental retardation, autism, and developmental delays, as well as behavior problems and gender-identity and eating disorders. Virtually any of the many types of problems that fall into these categories can be worsened by MTBI.

DIAGNOSING PSYCHIATRIC PROBLEMS

A trained professional can easily diagnose certain prior or underlying psychiatric disorders, such as schizophrenia or psychosis, as being separate from MTBI. However, this not the case with problems such as obsessive-compulsive disorder, mood disorders, and other psychiatric problems. Symptoms of these disorders can mimic those of other problems related to MTBI. It is therefore vital that your mental health care practitioner consider your preinjury personality as part of the diagnostic evaluation. A neuropsychological evaluation (see Chapter 2) is the best source of this information.

If you, a friend, or a family member suspects that you may have a psychological disorder that has been made worse by MTBI, you should consult with a psychiatrist or psychologist who specializes in brain injury and who can make the critical distinctions needed for correct diagnosis. Fatigue, for instance, can be an aftereffect of injury or a symptom of depression. Vague chronic pain can signal physical injury, injury in the area of the brain that perceives pain, somatoform disorder, malingering, or an emotional reaction. An experienced professional can conduct appropriate testing and assess substance abuse, behavior, denial, and other emotional reactions.

TREATING MTBI-RELATED PSYCHIATRIC PROBLEMS

There are a number of unique difficulties associated with the treatment of MTBI-related psychiatric problems. To begin with, because of the very nature of these problems, the first and most necessary step toward finding appropriate treatment—recognizing that something is wrong and that some type of help is needed—is often more difficult than it is with other types of disorders. Friends, family members, or coworkers often realize that there is a problem before the affected individual does, and it may take some time to convince him or her to accept the possibility. Then, too, in the past, many mental health professionals were hesitant to treat brain-injured people because they mistakenly believed that such people were unlikely to show significant improvement. In addition, little research has been done on treating patients with combined neurological and psychological problems. In fact, therapists trying to provide such treatment often experience many of the same emotions—especially frustration and hopelessness—that plague their patients.

Nevertheless, there are a number of conventional and alternative approaches to treating psychiatric disorders. Those that have been found to be the most successful for people with MTBI are described below.

Conventional Approaches

In general, psychiatric disorders respond best when traditional psychotherapy, cognitive-behavioral therapy, and, in some instances, EEG biofeedback are used along with appropriate medications. A psychopharmacologist (a psychiatrist who specializes in using drugs to treat psychiatric disorders) can work with you to determine the medication and dosage appropriate for your specific problem. Clinical depression is often best treated through a combination of psychotherapy and nonsedating antidepressant medications, such as fluoxetine (Prozac) or sertraline (Zoloft).

Chronic pain syndrome can be treated by a pain clinic (see the Resources list beginning on page 281), a rehabilitation hospital, or a psychologist who is board certified in behavioral medicine and has specialized in pain control. Biofeedback and hypnosis are also extremely effective against pain.

Substance abuse responds best to a combination of therapies, including twelve-step programs such as Alcoholics Anonymous (AA) or Narcotics Anonymous (NA) and behavior-modification psychotherapy. If you have a substance-abuse problem, it is extremely important for you to remember that an MTBI can make you more sensitive to any substance, making it difficult for you to tolerate the same doses of drugs or alcohol that you once consumed—or, in some cases, to tolerate any amount of these substances. Behavior modification is also useful for treating disruptiveness, compulsiveness, eating disorders, and other manifestations of emotional difficulty.

Alternative Approaches

Acupuncture and polarity therapy are extremely effective against chronic pain syndrome. These approaches can also be useful in the treatment of substance abuse and, in some cases, psychiatric disorders. Both acupuncture and polarity therapy should be performed by trained practitioners.

Certain over-the-counter herbal preparations and homeopathic remedies advertise that they can diminish depression, agitation, and other symptoms related to psychiatric disorders. Before you purchase any such product, it is important to realize that having both an MTBI and a psychiatric disorder creates an extremely complex situation. It is crucial to locate an herbalist or homeopathic practitioner who is willing to work with your psychopharmacologist and/or mental health professional (and vice versa). Such a team can properly evaluate your circumstances and specific needs, discuss types of products and dosages, and select the herbal or homeopathic remedies that are best for you. If your physician is unable to provide you with an appropriate referral, organizations such as the Herb Research Foundation and/or the National Center for Homeopathy (see the Resources section beginning on page 281) may be able to help.

PRACTICAL SUGGESTIONS

When it comes to psychiatric problems, treatment under the guidance of a mental health professional is the surest route to recovery. However, there are a number of things you can do to speed up the process on your own, and enhance your chances for a successful recovery. Here are some helpful ideas:

- Honestly acknowledge the fact that you have a problem and assume responsibility for it. Unless you do this, you will not be able to bring about the changes you need to get well.

- Insist upon working with a compassionate mental health professional who has an understanding of brain injury and its effect on psychiatric disorders.

- Join a self-help or support group. Your local hospital or community mental health center can put you in touch with the appropriate parties.

- Participate in group therapy with an understanding mental health professional.

- Seek on-line one-to-one support through computer bulletin boards.

- Be aware that help for people with chronic pain syndrome is becoming more widely available as hospitals and clinics recognize the need for such services.

- Consider seeking the comfort of a religious or spiritual group.

- Allow yourself to be receptive to the guidance and encouragement of family and friends.

While psychiatric problems can be very distressing, it can be reassuring to know that most individual symptoms are not physical effects of your MTBI. Instead, your injury has only heightened a pre-existing condition. Today, with consistent and proper medical and psychological care, most psychiatric problems are treatable. By finding the right approach and investing time and effort in recovery, you can significantly reduce the grip that psychiatric problems have on your life.

21

GRIEVING

In his youth, 52-year-old Jack had been a star in three sports: track, football, and baseball. After college and a stint in the Marines, he became a law-enforcement officer in Massachusetts, a job he held for over twenty-three years.

One June day, Jack was struck by a car and thrown over ten feet. He was unconscious for only a few minutes, and could recall everything about the accident by the time medical assistance arrived. At the local emergency room, the headache and dizziness Jack complained of were attributed to MTBI and postconcussive syndrome. Eventually, Jack was also diagnosed as having posttraumatic stress disorder.

Since his accident, Jack has repeatedly sought help for stuttering, fatigue, and depression. Several medical and mental health professionals have treated Jack for specific problems related to his MTBI, but he is still far from well. Now retired from the police force, Jack spends most of his days in bed. Even counseling by a priest has failed to improve his attitude toward his problems. Surprisingly, neither Jack's priest nor any of the specialists who have treated him has ever mentioned the possibility that his recovery has been stalled by grief over his loss of self.

Grieving is a normal process that relieves sorrow and allows us to adjust to loss. Many people think of grieving as something that happens only after certain specific events, such as the death of a loved one, but it occurs in response to other types of loss as well. For instance, as you grow older, you periodically mourn the loss of the younger person you once were. This is part of the process of adjusting to advancing age. If you experience a life-changing event like an MTBI, grieving the loss of the person you used to be is not only natural, but is actually a necessary part of recovery.

GRIEVING THE LOSS OF SELF

"In the past, I took my photographic memory for granted. In twenty years of doing psychotherapy, I never took notes during a session but, later, could recall every detail of the sessions that occurred that day. It is difficult to acknowledge that I have total amnesia to certain events that have occurred in my life. What I do know is that in one brief second on a beautiful March day, my previous life died."

—D.R.S.

The concept of *self* is complex. It is made up of two parts: the real self and the capacities of the self. According to psychologists, the structure of the real self consists of self-image (how you think of yourself), self-representation (how you present yourself), supraordiant self-organization (how you feel and present yourself over time), and the total self (who you really are). These aspects interact with each other. For example, you may think of yourself as a good worker, which may or may not be the case, and you may hope that others think so, too, which they or may not do. With the development of the real self come the capacities of the self, which include creativity, intimacy, aliveness, assertiveness, and commitment—all of which enable you to develop thoughts, be caring, feel enjoyment, and pursue your dreams.

The sense of self is not fully developed until adulthood. It is gained through work and through social relationships, especially family relationships and assuming the role of caretaker. At different points in your life, usually spurred by lifestyle, career, or physical changes, you will relinquish a former self-image and move on. This natural process can be drastically altered and/or accelerated by circumstances such as loss of employment, natural disaster, a close encounter with death, or a personal disaster.

An MTBI is experienced as a personal disaster. If your injury has robbed you of some of your ability to function at work or at home, this can have a crushing effect, because for most people, one's occupation is a prime source of purpose and gratification in life. In addition, you may feel less able to interact with your family, socialize, and pursue hobbies. After MTBI, you may have to face the possibility that you will never be as you once were. This experience constitutes a *loss of self*, and loss of self triggers grieving.

EXPERIENCING THE GRIEVING PROCESS

Healthy grieving can be more prolonged, pervasive, and complicated than you may realize. While not all grieving follows the same pattern, certain phases have been observed often enough to be recognized as typical. In most cases, the phases of grieving include the following:

- *Denial of the loss.* This phase includes being truly unaware of losses—or, in the case of MTBI, deficits. You may firmly believe that you are no different than before.

- *Anger.* This phase often manifests itself in expressions of rage and bouts of aggression over the injustice of the loss.

- *Bargaining.* Here, you try to set terms that will change the eventual outcome—as in, "If I do _____ [fill in the blank], things will be different."

- *Disorganization.* At this stage, you feel confused and have difficulty ordering your thoughts and behavior.

- *Despair.* This phase involves the loss of hope that things will ever be any better.

- *Depression.* Here, you experience emotions of hopelessness, inadequacy, and worthlessness. You may have eating and sleeping problems, exhibit anxious or withdrawn behavior, and even think of suicide.

- *Acceptance or resolution.* At this phase, you acknowledge your limitations and feel comfortable knowing that life can continue.

In the immediate aftermath of your injury, you may experience shock, numbness, or bewilderment. Emptiness, remorse, waves of crying, and attempts to regain what you have lost often follow in the ensuing weeks or months. Overall, you may feel sad and unable to experience pleasure—alternating, perhaps, with tense, restless anxiety. You may even notice one or more physical symptoms, such as sleep disturbances, loss of appetite, headaches, back pain, shortness of breath, heart palpitations, indigestion, dizziness, or nausea. In an attempt to prevent painful feelings, you may distance yourself emotionally from friends and family.

Clearly, grief has many depression-like symptoms (see Chapter 20), and depression can sometimes accompany grieving. A person experiencing normal, healthy grieving only, however, does not usually have the general feeling of worthlessness typical of a depressed person, and he or she may demonstrate episodes of lighter moods interspersed with depressed feelings—circumstances not seen in clinical depression. However, the depression-like symptoms of grieving can last as long as several years, until you can finally consider your loss without feeling overwhelming sadness, and you have begun to invest energy in other thoughts and activities.

Working through and letting go of grief is difficult, but it can be made less so by redirecting your energy to such activities as learning new skills, volunteering your services, or being a support person for another brain-injured individual. Gradually, you will begin to acknowledge and accept a new identity, which will allow your grief to fade into memory. However, if you merely stifle or obstruct your grief, the result may be pathological grief—a paralyzing sadness that lasts longer than a year, with no movement toward recovery from the loss. In most cases, pathological grief is characterized by continuing denial of reality or preoccupation with death and dying in general.

The greater your perceived loss of skills and abilities, the more extensive your sense of loss will be. Compulsively successful, high-achieving intellectual people, for instance, often experience a powerful loss of self if their thinking ability is even very slightly impaired. Very independent people, who are seen by others as leaders, caretakers, or sources of guidance, may be devastated if they become unable to live up to their previous self-reliant image. Young adults between the ages of eighteen and twenty-two are tremendously affected by grief after MTBI. Psychologists believe this is because at that age, a person has acquired a self-image, but has not yet had the opportunity to establish a sense of achievement or purpose. In contrast, older people have already enjoyed the accomplishment of some of their life goals and so tend to grieve less. Children also tend to be less affected by grief, probably because they are unable to recall functioning at another level. They therefore have less trouble blending MTBI-related deficits into their self-perception.

RECOGNIZING GRIEF

Grief over the loss of self is something every brain-injured person goes through. However, grieving often is not recognized for what it is because the resulting distractibility, anger, fatigue, and other signs can be masked by or confused with the symptoms of postconcussive syndrome or posttraumatic stress disorder. (*See* Identifying the Symptoms of Grief, page 219, for a comparison.) Also, lack of insight, which may make you unable to correctly evaluate the impact your symptoms are having on your life, is a typical aftereffect of MTBI. Unfortunately, the recognition of grief as a possible cause of postinjury behavior has eluded many physicians and mental-health professionals as well as MTBI survivors themselves. Many doctors tend to attribute symptoms of grief following an MTBI to the physical consequences of the injury.

Identifying the Symptoms of Grief

The process of grieving the loss of self that follows MTBI is often un-acknowledged, and its symptoms are often confused with those of post-concussive syndrome (PCS) or posttraumatic stress disorder (PTSD). The table below offers a comparison of the typical symptoms associated with these three conditions.

Symptom	Postconcussive Syndrome	Posttraumatic Stress Disorder	Healthy Grief
Amnesia	Yes	Yes	No
Anger	Yes	Yes	Yes
Lack of awareness	Yes	No	No
Concentration problems	Yes	Yes	Yes
Depression	Yes	Sometimes	Sometimes
Despair	Yes	Yes	Yes
Disorganization	Yes	Yes	Yes
Distractibility	Yes	Yes	Yes
Dizziness	Yes	Sometimes	Sometimes
Lack of emotion	Yes	Yes	No
Fatigue	Yes	Yes	Yes
Headaches	Yes	Sometimes	Sometimes
Isolation and withdrawal	Yes	Yes	Yes
Poor judgment	Yes	No	No
Nightmares, flashbacks	Yes	Yes	No
Personality changes	Yes	Yes	Sometimes
Attempts to regain previous self-image	Yes	Yes	Yes
Short-term memory loss	Yes	Yes	Sometimes
Sleep disturbances	Yes	Yes	Yes
Ultimate acceptance/ resolution	Yes	Yes	Yes

Understanding that there are emotional components to your loss of self is critical to winning family support and obtaining appropriate professional guidance. All too often, loved ones say things like "Control yourself," or "Think how lucky you are to be alive." They may mean well, but statements like these only perpetuate grief. The eventual resolution of your grieving can come only with sympathy, patience, the acknowledgment by you and by others that you are a different person than before—and, most important, with time.

Within the medical community, there is still much ground to be covered in this area. The idea of grieving following an MTBI has been largely overlooked by doctors; even the most highly trained psychotherapists sometimes may lack knowledge about brain injury, much less about grieving the resultant loss of self. It pays to keep looking, therefore, until you find a professional who understands the sadness and mourning you feel.

WORKING THROUGH YOUR GRIEF

"I often think of myself as a house that was hit by a hurricane and then restored. The MTBI destroyed portions of the house, which was me. The years of rehabilitation were like adding new lumber and materials onto the original design. To all appearances, the restored house is the same, but it is not. It is a composite of the old and the new. I look and sound similar to my old self, but I'm really a blend of the old and the new. In the years since my MTBI, I've done a lot of grieving, and I've finally learned to accept who I am now."
                                                                          —D.R.S.

Grieving is an emotionally painful but necessary part of life. Fortunately, there are a number of approaches that can assist you as you pass through the stages of the grief process. There are now therapists who specialize in grief work who can enable you to recognize and express your fear and sadness in a "safe" environment, without worrying about how your feelings may affect loved ones or how they might respond. Assisting rather than resisting grief will allow you to come to terms more quickly with your new situation.

Grief therapy is tailored to several variables, including developmental factors, the circumstances of your injury, your preinjury personality, and previous experiences you may have had with denial of your grief by support people in your life. Optimally, the therapist you choose should have previous experience working with patients grieving the loss of self due to injury (he or she need not have specific expertise in MTBI, however). Your doctor, a local rehabilitation facility, or the nearest Veterans' Administration hospital should be able to refer you to a qualified specialist. As with any mental health professional you choose to work with, it is important that you feel completely comfortable with your therapist.

On a practical, everyday level, simply recognizing and accepting the grieving process can do a great deal to make it easier to bear.

As you undergo the grieving process, you may find the following suggestions helpful:

- *Acknowledge the reality of your loss.* Ignore any express or implied messages from doctors, family, or friends to "snap out of it" or "get a grip." You cannot get on with your life until you grieve, and you cannot resolve your grief unless you recognize that your MTBI has made you a new person.

- *Identify and express your grief.* Therapy will help you to experience the pain and intense feelings that accompany the loss of self.

- *Commemorate your loss.* After the death of a loved one, the grieving process is aided by religious or cultural rituals and customs. Some people with MTBI have found it helpful to honor the memory of past accomplishments by collecting mementos of their old selves and burying them—whether literally or figuratively.

- *Acknowledge your ambivalence.* You may well have conflicting feelings about your MTBI. Sometimes you may view your survival as a second chance, while at other times you may see it as nothing but a burden. Such mixed feelings are normal, but if you do not recognize them, this inner conflict can pose a considerable barrier to the resolution of your grief. Instead of denying conflicting feelings, work toward a balance between positive and negative feelings about your new self and put them into perspective.

- *Learn to let go.* Ultimately, you must withdraw your emotional investment in the person you once were in order to go forward with your life. Realize that the person you are today is not a poor substitute, but a composite of your old and newly acquired selves.

- *Move on.* Resist viewing yourself as a tragic figure whom life has dealt a cruel blow. Relinquish plans and dreams that revolved around your former self and rethink your goals based on your present strengths and abilities.

While the recognition of your loss is a painful process, it is important to work toward emphasizing the good qualities you still possess. With guidance, you can bridge the gap between your pre- and postinjury selves, and emerge with strength, motivation, a redefined creative side, and a restored sense that life has meaning. It hurts to accept the reality that you may never completely recover, and both recovery and grieving can be slow processes. Once you give yourself permission to grieve, however, you will find the going much easier.

PART FIVE

RECOVERING

INTRODUCTION

George and Paula and their two children, Kevin and Susan, were involved in a five-car collision in Georgia. They underwent x-rays and CT scans at the local emergency room, all with negative results. In the weeks and months that followed, however, each was troubled by symptoms that included dizziness, headaches, memory problems, excessive fatigue, and difficulties with reading and concentration.

George, the first to seek help, was diagnosed with postconcussive syndrome, and was told to take a few weeks off from his job as a computer programmer. Paula, a second-grade teacher, also sought medical assistance, after she was told by her principal that her speech was unclear and that she seemed confused and disorganized. On a neurologist's advice, she took a leave of absence from work. Meanwhile, their children, tenth-grader Kevin and fifth-grader Susan, were having trouble at school. Their grades plummeted, and Kevin's behavior became quite aggressive. Susan seemed withdrawn and visibly depressed. Officials at both their schools recommended psychological evaluation and family counseling.

During the next three years, both George and Paula took early retirement from their jobs. The children's problems, which by now included substance abuse, also continued. They attempted therapy several times without success, and the future looked bleak—until Paula began to attend meetings of a brain-injury support group. Here, for the first time, she realized that many of her family's problems could be linked to their car accident, and that her lack of insight was probably a function of her own injury.

Five years after the accident, the family was reevaluated. A team of specialists developed rehabilitation programs for each family member, a step that turned their lives around within a year. George is now self-employed, Paula has returned to teaching, Kevin is a community-college student, and Susan is on the high-school honor roll. The family mourns the five years they lost, but, for the first time in many months, they can look forward to the future.

Recovery from mild traumatic brain injury is a complex process. Part Five of this book deals with different aspects of recovery, including rehabilitation, financial issues, the problems of living with someone with an MTBI, and MTBI outcomes. The path toward wellness may be a rocky one, but the information provided in the following chapters can make the going easier for you.

22

REHABILITATION

Randi, a 20-year-old Long Island college student, was on her way to meet a friend for dinner when, for no apparent reason, her car went out of control. Randi never really lost consciousness after the accident, but she remembers nothing about the first two weeks she spent in the hospital, bruised beyond recognition from her numerous physical injuries.

Randi underwent numerous CT scans, spinal taps, and EEGs before doctors reached a diagnosis of MTBI. When she was discharged after three weeks, Randi was paralyzed on one side of her face, blind in one eye, and deaf in one ear. She had significant memory loss and no sense of smell, and her right eye turned inward. No one knew the extent to which Randi might recover, yet she was not told that there were rehabilitation services that could help her. On her own, Randi pursued psychotherapy and medical assistance. With determination and the help of a wonderful support system, the young woman was able to return to college after only eight months. She made the dean's list and won a merit scholarship, and is now a graduate-school student. Recently, she married a long-time friend.

Not all people with MTBI are as fortunate as Randi. While this young woman and her family were able to focus their energies on her recovery, many people who have suffered such accidents lack the necessary direction, financial wherewithal, and family support to devote themselves to recovery. Instead, they may be left with an innocent-sounding diagnosis, unexpected problems at home and on the job, and little or no information about programs that can help them live a quality life once again.

The Brain Injury Association uses the motto, "Life after head injury may never be the same." However, the right rehabilitation program can take you a long way toward recovery.

WHY REHABILITATION SERVICES ELUDE MANY PEOPLE WITH MTBI

"Despite the fact that one of my neurologists is based in a rehabilitation facility with a mild traumatic brain injury section, and another is located near a hospital with an entire inpatient unit for MTBIs, I realized only recently that coordinated rehabilitation services were available to me. After my accident, I was treated with various outpatient therapies, and I was making progress. But then I had a setback that left me with right-side weakness, slurred speech, poor judgment, problems with thinking and remembering, and intense pain in my right arm, shoulder, neck, and upper back. After lengthy testing, a neuropsychologist asked if I would consider rehabilitation. In fact, he was amazed that none of my previous doctors had ever suggested this service or informed me that it existed for people with my type of injury. Now that I know, I'm exploring new avenues to ensure my ongoing recovery."

—D.R.S.

Recent estimates indicate that there are over 700 brain-injury rehabilitation programs nationwide. Services of this type are standard procedure for people who suffer moderate or severe head injuries. In fact, most such people are referred directly from the hospital. Many people with MTBI do not require hospitalization, however, and those who do are usually admitted for treatment of bodily injuries only. As a result, the symptoms of brain injury, which may surface one at a time, are most often addressed on an outpatient basis—sometimes by several different doctors, and often by doctors who lack training in the complexities of this type of injury.

Overall, a person with an MTBI is frequently left to piece together his or her own recovery program—a process that can be significantly hampered by some of the very skill deficits that make rehabilitation necessary, such as difficulties with organization, memory, and judgment. Do-it-yourself rehabilitation can certainly be successful, but it lacks the cohesiveness and sense of security offered by a coordinated team approach.

WHY REHABILITATION MAY BE NECESSARY AFTER MTBI

Not all MTBI patients require rehabilitation. It may be that outpatient treatment of symptoms is enough to bring about marked improvement and enable you to return to work and other everyday activities within a reasonable period of time. On the other hand, you may find that your job performance and daily living skills are so greatly affected by MTBI that changes in your daily routine are necessary. Or you may be so consumed by the aftereffects of your injury that your life lacks fulfillment. You may suffer chronic pain, debilitating fatigue, or have specific impairments that just are not improving.

If any of these is the case, the team approach adopted by many rehabilitation hospitals may be the best means of improving your quality of life. Rehabilitation may involve working on an outpatient basis with one or more of the following specialists: a neurologist, a neuropsychologist, a physiatrist, a psychologist, a physical therapist, an occupational therapist, a speech/language pathologist, and a vocational therapist. In facilities that have pain units, pain-management techniques may also be taught.

A good place to start when looking for a rehabilitation program is the Commission for Accreditation of Rehabilitation Facilities (CARF) (see the Resources section at the end of the book), which can direct you to the nearest facility that offers team services for outpatients. Otherwise, you will probably have to piece together a program on your own, a task that can be overwhelming.

FINDING THE RIGHT REHABILITATION PROGRAM

Rehabilitation programs available for people with MTBI vary. In some localities, there are specific mild traumatic brain injury units; in others, you might be eligible for vocational rehabilitation, counseling, and/or physical or occupational therapy services. Getting into an appropriate program is not always easy. Although federal regulations prohibit the use of a patient's age as a factor in determining eligibility for rehabilitation services, there have been instances in which people have been turned away from programs because of their age. Many programs have long waiting lists, and some have residency requirements. In addition, you may be refused admission to a program if it is determined that your disability does not substantially handicap your daily living or job skills, or that rehabilitation services will not improve your employability. Most rehabilitation programs require some evidence (from the type of injury and your initial moves toward recovery) that your condition is likely to improve.

Medical insurance coverage may also be a factor. Some insurance companies will pay for participation only in rehabilitation programs that have contractual arrangements with them. If you are in a managed-care plan, it is helpful—indeed, it may be necessary—to get your primary-care physician to assist you in getting into an appropriate re-habilitation program.

Before you sign up for any rehabilitation program, you should become as informed as possible about all aspects of the program and the services offered. *See* Factors to Consider When Comparing Rehabilitation Programs, page 231, for suggested questions to ask to help you evaluate rehabilitation programs.

Whatever your particular circumstances, it is wise to remember that rehabilitation is time-consuming and requires a strong physical and emotional commitment. Just as you might seek a second medical opinion, it is advisable to shop around for the program best suited to your specific needs. After all, different programs have different success rates in different skill areas. The following suggestions can help you take an active role in this important part of your recovery:

- Have a diagnostic assessment done to determine which of three major areas—physical, mental, and emotional capabilities—require rehabilitation.

- Ask your neurologist or neuropsychologist for program recommendations. (Be aware, though, that you and your doctor may differ in your opinions as to the necessity of rehabilitation.)

- Ask for program referrals from your disability or insurance company.

- Contact the Brain Injury Association to determine whether your state has its own brain-injury organization. Request referrals from both groups.

- Visit recommended facilities in person. Do not rely on brochures or telephone descriptions.

- Ask to speak to families who have used the programs you are considering (but remember that facilities will likely offer names of satisfied customers only).

- Consider both nearby facilities and more distant ones. Location may be a factor if you cannot drive, but transportation arrangements can often be made if a faraway program is better suited to your needs.

- If your insurance company limits your choice of facilities, explore the possibility of using a nonparticipating facility anyway, if you feel strongly that it is the best for you. Insurance companies occasionally do extend coverage to outside programs. If your request is refused, ask the facility about working out a reasonable payment program.

Factors to Consider When Comparing Rehabilitation Programs

The goal of rehabilitation is to enable you to resume your normal every-day activities. You will make the most rapid progress toward this goal if the program you choose is a good fit for you and your needs. The following are some questions to ask when considering a rehabilitation program:

- Will rehabilitation be done on a one-to-one or group basis? *Depending on your diagnosis, a combination of the two may be better than one or the other.*

- Are the members of the interdisciplinary team full-time staff members or consultants? *People who are supervised by personnel within the hospital are best.*

- Will more than one therapist or team member be working on my program? *The team approach is preferable as a means of getting a full range of care.*

- How often would I have to go to the facility? *Your allowed number of days of rehabilitation services may be limited by your insurance coverage.*

- Who would make decisions about my progress? *Ideally, the team and program manager or rehabilitation physician will make decisions at team meetings, aided by the patient and family members.*

- What is the cost of the program? *It is wise to compare the costs of comparable programs.*

- Is transportation provided by the facility for outpatient services? If so, what type is available? Are there mileage limitations?

- Does this facility offer all of the services that are recommended for my care, including speech, vocational, educational, physical, and/or occupational therapy, as well as psychotherapy and case management? If not, can they contract out to other outpatient service providers?

- Is case management available for both inpatient and outpatient treatment? *This service can be extremely important to the success of your rehabilitation.*

> The answers to these questions will help you to determine which fa-
> cilities are best suited to your needs. It is very important for you and
> a trusted friend or family member to make personal visits to programs
> under consideration, rather than making decisions based only on tele-
> phone interviews. Once you have chosen the right facility for your sit-
> uation, ask to see the Patients' Rights list published by that facility. Use
> this information to help yourself. Many institutions also have lending
> libraries that afford access to books, articles, audiotapes, and videos about
> MTBI.

- Be aware that home rehabilitation programs exist for people who
  are immobile. The Brain Injury Association can help you locate such
  a program.

- Attend local brain-injury support groups and ask whether other
  members have been in rehabilitation. Ask for details about any programs you learn of.

- If you are receiving workers' compensation, let your case manager
  take an active role in getting you the help you need. Remember,
  he or she wants you to return to work successfully.

It can take as long as two to three months to determine your specific rehabilitation needs and locate the most suitable program, but
this is time well spent. The uniqueness of every MTBI and the many
personal circumstances that can affect recovery make the selection of
your program a most important decision.

MANAGING THE REHABILITATION PROCESS

*"Four years after my accident, I tried the Burdenko method of water thera-
py. It did for me what four years of weights, Nautilus training, swimming,
aquatherapy, medication, and alternative treatments had not been able to do:
It enabled me to negotiate stairs without pain, kneel without falling, walk
without staggering, and begin to rebuild lost muscle tone. In fact, a few
months of the Burdenko method put me back on my bicycle for the first time
since my accident."*

—D.R.S.

When you enroll in a rehabilitation program, you should be assigned
a case manager to coordinate your insurance and medical care, and
to work with your lawyer when needed to seek reimbursement for
costs not covered by insurance. If your job skills have been severely

affected by your MTBI, you may also be assigned a counselor to assist you in reentering the job market.

Diagnostic assessments will be required by any rehabilitation program you choose. Your test results will help specialists pinpoint the exact services that are needed. If you have had previous testing done on an outpatient basis, you may be able to save time, money, and needless duplication of tests by providing the rehabilitation facility with these records. Home and workplace assessments may also be done to evaluate your support system and see whether changes are needed in your physical environment. Then a personalized program will be developed according to test and assessment results. Therapists will be assigned, and specific goals and time frames will be defined. Be aware that there may be skills that cannot be regained through rehabilition. If this proves to be the case, you will be taught other ways to do these things, as well as methods of coping with your limitations.

It is important to get to know the people involved with your case. Communication between you and the various specialists, and between the specialists and your outpatient doctors, will help you achieve your goals more quickly. Sometimes, home instruction may be advised, either at the hands of a staff member or a friend or family member who has been trained by the rehabilitation team.

Your team can also assist your employer or school system in making adaptations designed to improve your effectiveness on the job or in the classroom. The Americans With Disabilities Act requires employers to make reasonable adaptations to allow disabled persons to work. For instance, an occupational therapist can help set up an appropriate work site and get a computer programmer to make a special program to suit the writing needs of a person with MTBI.

Naturally, there are a vast number of rehabilitative approaches that may be used. The appropriate techniques vary from patient to patient. The formulation of your rehabilitation program will be based on your specific needs. It may include speech and language therapy to improve communication skills; occupational therapy to help with organizational skills; physical therapy to improve mobility; and psychological services to help you cope with all of the changes that have taken place in your life. Some rehabilitation programs provide driver-evaluation programs to assess your physical and emotional readiness to resume driving.

Rehabilitation programs are meant to help you resume a normal daily life after significant injury. While rehabilitation is not always necessary after MTBI, and may not even come up in consultations with your primary-care physician, these types of programs and specialists do exist to help you. In many cases, the right rehabilitation program can eliminate confusion, minimize frustration, and accelerate your recovery process.

23

FINANCIAL ISSUES

Valerie, whose story appears in the Introduction to Part Three, lives in Maryland, a state whose insurance laws mandate a minimum of five thousand dollars in personal injury protection (PIP) for every driver. This insurance is meant to cover the policyholder's initial medical expenses in the event of an automobile accident. The assumption is that an injured party can sue to recover expenses above that amount if necessary. Valerie—like most of the 98 percent of Marylanders who purchase only minimum PIP coverage—never considered that the five thousand dollars might be inadequate. She discovered this only after her accident. Valerie also didn't realize that being injured in an accident might make it impossible for her to obtain medical insurance—until a sharp premium increase forced her to cancel an existing medical policy after her accident. For three years, she was repeatedly denied replacement coverage, until a lawyer suggested that she purchase open-enrollment insurance. This is a costly and very limited type of hospitalization and catastrophe coverage that cannot be denied to anyone, regardless of preexisting conditions. Valerie says that the benefits provided by this policy are a disappointment, but at least it covers most catastrophic hospital bills—a concern due to her family medical history.

Valerie sees herself as a victim of the auto accident that ended her artistic career, and also as a victim of the legal and health-care systems that were supposed to help her. She is lucky to have a family that has been able to assist her financially. Even so, she has at times thought about moving with her husband to his native Italy, where the government-run health-care system would afford her better care than she has received in the United States.

MTBI carries with it two main financial issues: lost wages due to layoff, firing, or a change in employment; and medical bills for the extensive services that are often needed after an injury of this type. This chapter examines both of these issues and gives advice concerning the types of financial help that may be available to you, as well as suggestions for dealing with reductions in income and tips to help you cut through the red tape that so often surrounds the insurance process.

LOST WAGES

Obviously, after an injury like MTBI, a certain recovery period is usually required before you can return to work. In some job situations, it is possible to take a medical leave of absence with pay. In others, you may be paid during your recuperation from illness or injury only to the extent of accumulated sick and vacation time. If you are self-employed or have no employer-provided benefits, you may not be able to get any paid time off at all.

Regardless of your employment situation, you may attempt to return to work during your recovery only to discover that your ability to function on the job is not what it was prior to injury. You may see the need to take a different job that calls for less intellectual processing, for example, or you may even have to stop working—at least for the present. Many people with MTBI end up losing their jobs because their work performance doesn't measure up after what their employers consider a "reasonable" period of time. Others leave voluntarily or abandon a business rather than face daily frustration and embarrassment.

The result is that many people with MTBI find themselves earning less money after injury than before. Meanwhile, normal household expenses remain more or less constant and medical bills mount up rapidly. Because it is often impossible to predict how fully you will recover from MTBI, or how long recovery will take, it is important to know how you can obtain financial compensation to help you with your expenses.

TYPES OF COMPENSATION

"Before my accident, I had a successful two-office psychology practice. Fortunately, I carried overhead insurance to cover fixed expenses such as rent, utilities, phone bills, advertising, managerial and secretarial help, and my answering service. I had income disability insurance and, because I was also an employee of my corporation, workers' compensation coverage. My overhead insurance covered my business expenses until I was able to close my offices, and, because my accident occurred as I was returning to my home office from visiting a patient, I also qualified for workers' compensation benefits. I was required to undergo four separate neuropsychological examinations and sever-

al consultations with an independent physician, but for the first four years, the workers' compensation agency was cooperative, congenial, and efficient. Then policy and personnel changes brought a rude awakening. Bills were delayed for months and then paid only in part, many more evaluations and tests were required, and my new claims representative hinted that many of my expenses would no longer be covered. I was forced to seek legal counsel."

—D.R.S.

The possibility of compensation for lost wages and medical bills is determined by the circumstances of your MTBI. As you read in Chapter 1, these injuries most commonly result from auto accidents, sports mishaps, falls, blows to the head, or assault. If your MTBI occurred in a car accident, financial support may be provided through automobile insurance. If your injury happened on the job, you can seek assistance through workers' compensation. Liability and health insurance usually cover sports and other injuries that take place on school premises; homeowner's insurance, health insurance, or, in some cases, government assistance may cover injuries that happen at home. Some states have victims' compensation laws that provide for financial assistance for persons injured as a result of physical assault.

Dealing with insurance companies and/or government agencies can be one of the most difficult and frustrating aspects of an MTBI. Payment for injury is a billion-dollar business that employs thousands of doctors, attorneys, investigators, consultants, and office personnel. When you become involved in this system, you become a case number in a huge maze. It is important to bear in mind that just because you have been the victim of a traumatic brain injury, you do *not* have to become a victim of bureaucracy and corporate decisions. Remember that insurance companies are in business to make a profit, and that these institutions deal daily with people who want to take advantage of the system. As you pursue your case, you are likely to encounter delays, tremendous amounts of paperwork, and a certain lack of sensitivity to your needs, so it is important to enlist someone—a family member, a trusted friend, or someone from your local brain-injury association—to be a personal advocate who will work with you on your behalf. In addition, it is often advisable to secure the services of an attorney. (*See* Finding the Right Attorney, page 238, for help in your search for appropriate legal counsel.) In this section, we will look at the various possibilities for financial compensation.

Automobile Insurance

Automobile insurance is designed to deal with responsibility, liability, and medical aspects of a car accident. In some states, a determina-

Finding the Right Attorney

It is often advisable to hire an attorney to help you through the process of securing compensation for your injury. Without legal help, this process may be exceptionally difficult for a person with MTBI, who looks fine but whose poor judgment places him or her at an enormous disadvantage before the process is even started.

To help locate an attorney with expertise in MTBI, ask your state brain-injury association if they have a referral list, or ask your health-care professional for help. If you are in a brain-injury support group, ask other members whose services they have used or whom they would recommend. Be cautious of lawyers who advertise on television. Claims of experience with injury cases are no guarantee that an attorney is necessarily the right choice for you.

Depending on where you live, you might be able to locate more than a few lawyers who are specialists in personal injury or workers' compensation and who have an understanding of traumatic brain injury. Once you have compiled a list, you should arrange to interview each candidate personally. This is extremely important, not only to ascertain a prospective lawyer's expertise but also to ensure that you feel comfortable with him or her. Because your MTBI may cause you to have problems recalling information, consider bringing a tape recorder, note pad, or friend or family member to the interview.

The following are questions to ask an attorney that can help you determine whether he or she has the background necessary to properly represent you after an MTBI:

- How many cases similar to mine have you been involved with as the principal attorney over the past three years? *Though the numbers may vary, it is important that the lawyer has had MTBI clients for whom he or she has won settlements.*

- What percentage of your practice is devoted to cases and injuries similar to mine? *This too may vary, depending on where you live, but it can be a good indication of an attorney's experience with MTBI cases.*

- What were the results in terms of settlements or verdicts in the last five cases that you handled involving injuries similar to mine?

- Could you furnish a list of prior MTBI clients?

- How many seminars or conferences have you attended over the past two years involving presentations on injuries similar to mine? *Ideally, your lawyer will have attended more than two such seminars.*

- How many articles have you written over the past three years involving any aspect of injury similar to mine? *It is desirable for your chosen attorney to have written at least one.*

- Would you explain the process you follow in handling a case like mine?

- Do you have consultants with expertise in MTBI?

- What kinds of problems might occur in the settlement process?

- Will you personally work on my case or do you have an assistant? If an assistant will be used, does that person have experience with MTBI?

- Will you personally be representing me in court? If not, who will? Does that person have expertise in MTBI?

- What are your legal fees? *Generally there are three types of fee arrangements: hourly fees, flat fees, and contingency fees. In most states, lawyers obtain a contingency fee—usually 33 percent—for auto accidents, and a fixed rate for workers' compensation settlements. The client does not pay the lawyer; rather, payment is received by the lawyer only if the client is awarded a monetary settlement.*

Following an MTBI, your choice of legal representation can be crucial to obtaining appropriate financial compensation for your injuries. Time invested in locating an experienced attorney will be time well spent.

tion must be made as to who was responsible for causing an accident before a claim for compensation can be settled. Traditionally, damages are paid by the insurer of the party determined to be at fault. Many states have sought to simplify this process by passing so-called "no-fault" insurance laws. Under no-fault insurance, each person's policy covers expenses incurred. If it can be established that one party is more than 50 percent at fault in the accident, his or her insurance company then assumes full financial responsibility.

There are three types of damage compensation that you may qualify for after an auto accident:

1. Special damages. These provide reimbursement for your medical expenses and compensation for lost wages.

2. General damages. These reimburse for what you could have earned if you had not been injured, and provide compensation for emotional pain and suffering caused in your daily life.

3. Punitive damages. Punitive damages may be assigned by the court if an insurance company fails to issue a reasonable settlement on a valid claim.

Most automobile-insurance policies have liability coverage to protect against both bodily and property damage. This will pay for damages you may cause someone else. If you live in a state with no-fault laws, you may have personal injury protection (PIP), which can cover both loss of wages and medical payments. In states with fault-based insurance laws, there is a similar type of coverage called MedPay for medical bills. Your insurance agent can provide specifics about the coverage afforded by your policy. Depending on where you live, you may also be able to purchase additional insurance to protect yourself against accident or injury caused by an uninsured motorist.

Following an accident, your first step should be to call your insurance agent—the same day, if possible. If you have sustained injuries from an auto accident and it is clearly not your fault, the insurance company will assign one of its own lawyers to act in your behalf. In many situations, if the details of what happened are clear-cut, you do not need to obtain your own lawyer. In other cases, your insurance company will advise you to do so. Most claims for medical compensation, suffering, and the like are negotiated between the insurance companies or settled out of court between lawyers. If your or the other party's insurance company questions the circumstances of an accident, it is imperative that you obtain private counsel.

Have your attorney and your personal advocate look at any proposed settlement with your or the other party's insurance company before you agree to it. Remember that symptoms do not always arise immediately after MTBI and that your injury may have affected your judgment.

Health Insurance

If your MTBI occurred as a result of a fall or sports injury, your medical expenses may be covered under your health-insurance policy. The extent of payment depends on the type of policy you have, the coverage it provides, and the amount of mandatory copayments, if any.

Many policies require you to choose doctors and medical facilities from among those participating in the health plan, which may mean choosing among health-care providers who lack specific training or experience in treating MTBIs. In most situations, health-insurance companies resist paying for care provided by practitioners outside their own networks, even though this can have a negative effect on the recovery process. However, a health-maintenance organization or preferred-provider association may allow outside consultations if you can prove that your health needs cannot be met otherwise.

The first step in arranging for care outside your health-plan network is to consult your primary-care physician. If he or she agrees that there is no one in the managed-care network to help you, then he or she should make a referral to an appropriate person outside the network. If your primary-care doctor refuses to make an outside referral because he or she will be penalized financially for doing so, you can see a doctor of your own choosing. In this situation, however, you will have to pay the outside doctor's cost yourself. You should then consult with your lawyer about including this bill in your settlement.

Available coverage and services usually depend on the health coverage you or your employer held prior to your accident, or what is covered under workers' compensation or the other party's policy. Some policies cover occupational therapy, chiropractic, and psychological services; some do not, or have strict limits on such coverage. Only in the past few years has alternative insurance that covers such services as acupuncture become available.

Government Programs

There are a number of different government programs that may provide benefits to people with MTBI: Medical Assistance (formerly called Medicaid); Medicare; Social Security Disability; Supplemental Security Income (SSI); and Veterans' Administration programs.

Medical Assistance is a combination state- and federally-funded program. Eligibility depends on your financial and medical needs. Depending on your state, there may be restrictions on coverage, including the types of treatment, equipment, and medication covered. Medicare pays for medical services for persons who are age sixty-five or older, or who have received Social Security Disability income (see below) for at least two years.

Social Security Disability (SSD) is available to individuals whose disability occurred within five years of their last employment and who were employed for a required period of time. If you are a

widow or widower and have become disabled, you may be eligible
for this benefit if your deceased spouse would have met the employment criteria. There is no set salary or income required for this
benefit. If you do not qualify for SSD, you and your dependents may
be eligible for the Supplemental Security Income (SSI) program. This
program is available to individuals with disabilities who have never
been employed or who became disabled before they contributed to
the Social Security fund through employment for a sufficient amount
of time. It is also available to those with little income and few resources.

If you need help in applying for any of these government benefits, call your local Social Security office, listed in the government section of your local telephone directory. They can give you guidance
and assistance in the application process. However, you should be
aware that getting this type of help can be difficult and time-consuming, and that eligibility requirements for certain benefits are subject to change in the future—most likely in the direction of becoming more restrictive. Nevertheless, you should not be discouraged if
your claim is rejected at first. With your doctor's support, persistence,
and an appeal or two, you may ultimately succeed in obtaining benefits.

In most states, there are Veterans' Administration hospitals with
physicians on staff who are knowledgeable about brain injuries. If you
served in the armed forces and have become disabled, you may be
eligible for wage or medical assistance. Contact the nearest office of
the Veterans' Administration, listed in the government section of your
local telephone directory, to determine whether you qualify and learn
how to apply.

In addition to these nationwide programs, some states also have
programs available to injured people who are eighteen years of age
or younger. Your local brain-injury association can advise you of state
programs for which you may be eligible. If you are disabled and have
minor children living at home, you may qualify for benefits under
Temporary Assistance for Needy Families. This program is adminis-
tered through the states and different states have different names for
it. Eligibility requirements and benefits likewise vary from state to
state. For specific information about benefits that may be available to
you and how to apply for them, contact your social services department.

One thing is more or less constant when dealing with any government agency: Getting adequate care can be difficult because you
must meet stringent requirements and deal with a fair amount of red
tape and paperwork in order to benefit from government programs.

In addition, the coverage provided is limited. In some states, outpatient services in particular are strictly limited. If you encounter problems filling out Medical Assistance or Medicare claims, you or your personal advocate can contact other doctors and medical facilities, a social-service worker, or your state legal-aid service for help in expediting your claim.

Workers' Compensation

"About ten years ago, I got a job as an assistant to a film director and his actress wife. Six years later, while checking the gate where I worked, I fell down onto the driveway. I was taken to the local hospital. My apparent injuries were two teeth protruding through my upper lip. In the weeks that followed, I experienced various symptoms of MTBI, such as smelling phantom smells, feeling cold, and having problems with articulation, memory loss, confusion, and poor judgment. I was contacted by a workers' compensation representative who suggested I see a neurologist. My doctor diagnosed me as having postconcussive syndrome. The claims person at workers' compensation suggested that I go home and rest. After a month, I felt better and attempted to resume working. However, I soon discovered that I could no longer perform the needed duties. I eventually quit my job.

In the years that have followed, I have been assigned several claims adjusters; however, no treatment was provided for my MTBI. I finally realized that I needed to hire an attorney to represent me. After years of waiting, I recently had neuropsychological testing done, but I am still awaiting appropriate rehabilitative treatment for my MTBI.

—Missy

If your MTBI was employment related, you are probably covered by workers' compensation laws. The time and procedure for filing varies from state to state, and the process itself can be tiresome and frustrating, so it is advisable to contact an attorney or a brain-injury association advocacy program for assistance. Under workers' compensation law, you may be entitled to receive a percentage of your preinjury earnings as well as payment for medical expenses. Before being approved for benefits, you will probably be required to undergo an evaluation by a specific medical professional under contract to the workers' compensation insurance carrier. This person's opinion may determine whether certain services will be covered and/or if existing services should be continued. If the insurance carrier's physician feels that particular services are not necessary, the carrier may stop paying for those services. If you disagree with the doctor's evaluation, you can get a second opinion and go to court to argue your side. Meanwhile, if you need the service under dispute, you must pay for it yourself or run up a bill.

Even payment for treatment approved under workers' compensation can be delayed, sometimes for long periods. It is not unusual for doctors to refuse to accept workers' compensation patients because of the paperwork, minimal payment, and other obstacles. Don't give up, however. Your local brain-injury association should be able to help you locate a qualified practitioner or practitioners who accept such patients.

Victims' Compensation

If your MTBI occurred as a result of a crime or physical assault, you may be entitled to compensation for lost wages and medical expenses through a state victims' compensation fund. Your lawyer, the local legal-aid society, or the office of your state's attorney can tell you whether there is such a fund in your state. The rules and requirements for receiving compensation from victims' funds differ, but in most states, a claim must be filed within a specified period of time. It is therefore important to find out what is needed and to get the necessary forms filled out as soon after your injury as possible.

Disability Insurance

Many companies supply income or disability insurance as part of an employee benefit package. Disability coverage pays a percentage of your previous wages while you are disabled, though exactly what percentage and for how long depends on the individual policy. The maximum dollar amount is not likely to approach the amount you previously earned, but it can help if you are unable to work. If you have this kind of coverage, your employer can advise you of the proper filing procedure. If you are self-employed and have private disability coverage, you will have to file a claim with the insurance company on your own. You may want to ask a family member or your attorney to work on your behalf to obtain the needed compensation.

PRACTICAL SUGGESTIONS

"I have saved a lot of time and energy by filling out the personal data section at the top of a blank medical form and then making photocopies of the entire form so that only the date and signature need to be added in the future."

—*Rita*

"I highly recommend learning to interview professionals to ensure that you are seeking help from appropriate sources. Also, make photocopies of every application, form, and cover page that you submit to agencies and insurance companies. If you need to reapply or be recertified for benefits in the future, you can simply copy the previous form."

—Elaine

"I'm fortunate in that I had insurance, and that I'm able to afford my daily bills—unlike many people with MTBI, who have to choose between paying medical bills and feeding their families. To help me cope with seemingly uncaring bureaucratic personnel, I've found comfort within my local brain-injury support group and from my psychotherapist and the many caring friends I've made in cyberspace.

—D.R.S.

The process of filing for compensation for lost wages and medical expenses can be long and frustrating. The suggestions that follow can make things a bit easier:

- Be organized. Keep a daily diary, beginning with the events that led to your injury. Keep all your medical records in one file, and create another file for records regarding your accident. List names of witnesses, emergency personnel, and doctors, and keep detailed notes about your symptoms. If necessary, ask a friend or family member for assistance with this.

- Document all telephone conversations relating to your accident by keeping a log. Include the date and time of each conversation, the name of the individual you spoke to, and a summary of your conversation.

- If you hire a lawyer to help you secure compensation for your injury, send him or her copies of your telephone log and all written correspondence relating to your accident and its aftermath. If your lawyer does the paperwork, keep notes of (or tape-record, with permission) your conversations with him or her.

- Find a good mental health therapist who has had experience with MTBI. If your health and recovery begin to be affected by your experiences with health-care providers, insurance companies, and government agencies, talk to your therapist about this.

- If strained finances prevent you from locating a mental health therapist, contact your local brain-injury association or a nearby hospital's mental health clinic for assistance.

- Seek out a support group. Call the Brain Injury Association (BIA) to see whether there is an MTBI group in your area. Also find out whether the BIA can put you in touch with an advocate to assist you with money issues.

- If you have access to a computer, explore on-line chat lines and bulletin boards. Discussing your problems with other people with MTBI can be extremely helpful. If you do not own a computer, check to see if your local public library has available for patrons computers with on-line capability.

Some people with MTBI may neither have insurance nor qualify for government compensation or assistance programs. It may be that your employer does not offer health insurance or other benefits, or perhaps you are self-employed, and you cannot or choose not to buy disability or medical insurance on your own because it simply costs too much. You may have lost your job after suffering an MTBI, and with it, your insurance—just when you needed it most. Or you may be able to work part time, but even though you do not qualify for employer-provided benefits, you earn too much to qualify for government assistance. Meanwhile, your household and medical bills continue to pile up. While a long-term solution may seem elusive, there are a few options to consider in these circumstances:

- Switch roles with your spouse. If you are the breadwinner, discuss the possibility of your spouse taking on more work hours or, perhaps, a second job.

- Change your lifestyle. Do what you can to prevent your household bills from becoming unmanageable, including selling your home or other assets if necessary. If needed, ask a trusted family member or friend to do an overall budget inventory to see what you are actually spending on things. Then you can discuss ways to scale back your spending and develop a reasonable budget to live on.

- Be honest about your situation with creditors, doctors, and your landlord or mortgage banker. You may be able to negotiate payment plans that are easier to meet.

- Allow friends and family to help. Doing so can be embarrassing, but accepting heartfelt assistance can help you through a very difficult time.

- Consider living with your parents, in-laws, or other willing relatives for an established period of time.

- If your children require assistance, contact your local mental health facility about free counseling and other services in your area.

- Contact your state chapter of the Brain Injury Association. Laws are always changing, and new options for financial assistance may become open to you. In addition to providing advocacy and other services, the BIA monitors such developments.

- Check with religious organizations in your community about funds and services available to people in need. They may offer or know of sources of basic necessities such as food and clothing at no or reduced cost.

- Ask your doctor or advocate about programs for obtaining prescription medications at reduced prices. Some pharmaceutical manufacturers offer such benefits to qualified persons.

- If you need a lawyer, check with your local and state government about free legal services available to people who qualify. Also, some attorneys dedicate a certain amount of their time to offering free, or *pro bono*, legal services. In some situations, these arrangements may not be necessary, since legal fees are usually collected as part of a settlement.

- Consult your bank about services that can advise you about managing your money and obtaining credit while you recover.

- If your financial situation is truly unmanageable, consider filing for personal bankruptcy. This decision should probably be considered a last resort, and it should be made with great care and under an attorney's guidance. However, bankruptcy can sometimes be the right choice, particularly if your debt is overwhelming.

Financial concerns are a very real part of coping with MTBI. The way money issues are dealt with can dramatically affect your final outcome. Not only do you need money for daily living expenses, but after MTBI, you are likely to need money to finance a rehabilitation process that can last for some time—in some cases, for years. It is not always easy to navigate the maze of red tape and paperwork required, but help is available to most people with MTBI through commercial insurance, health insurance, government assistance, workers' compensation, and victims' compensation. When coping with monetary difficulties, it helps to remember that you are not alone. Consult with trusted family members or friends, an attorney with expertise in MTBI, and/or your local brain-injury association, and allow yourself to accept their advice and assistance.

24

LIVING WITH SOMEONE WITH AN MTBI

Jeff, the husband of Gail from Chapter 4, says that living with a person with MTBI takes patience . . . patience . . . patience, because the person you love isn't the same anymore. Jeff describes his wife as an incredible person who used to give 120 percent to her work, her family, and making a home. She was consistent and dependable, and very tolerant and understanding. The impact of Gail's injury on the family—their daughters were five and three years old at the time—was like someone turning off the lights, Jeff says. The unpredictability of her symptoms, the frequency and extent of her anger, and her difficulty handling more than one activity at a time are what cause him and the children the most frustration. For a long time, the older daughter wouldn't admit that Gail had been in a car accident. She is now getting psychological help, as well as support from Jeff's parents, who live nearby and help out often. The younger daughter also has been traumatized.

Jeff estimates that Gail has now returned to 85 percent of her old self. She has taken a job as a crossing guard and is gradually exhibiting more normal behavior. But the family has to live with the unpredictability of Gail's symptoms and eventual outcome, and that takes patience . . . patience . . . patience.

An MTBI affects everyone whose life is touched by the injured person, particularly family and friends. How these important people are affected, and the way in which they respond, can affect the individual's recovery process and eventual outcome.

EMOTIONAL RESPONSES

My family loves me for what I was, and protects what I am.
My friends cherish what I was, and often forget what I am.
I remember who I was. I want to find out who I am.
It is now ten o'clock. At least I know where I am.

These first lines from Beverley Bryant's poem "From Inside Out" tell of the conflict family and friends have in dealing with MTBI. If a loved one suffers such an injury, you can expect to undergo a series of reactions that are similar to the classic stages of grief, from denial to anger to depression to ultimate acceptance of the new reality. Of course, not everyone goes through the same reactions in the same order, or wrestles with each one for the same amount of time. Also, it is possible to experience two or more of these reactions simultaneously. As a general rule, however, friends and family members of a person with MTBI can expect to experience something like the progression of emotional responses outlined below.

Denial

"To my three teenaged sons, nothing has changed since my accident except my unpredictability. They often complain about never knowing when I won't be feeling well or what will cause me to lose my temper. I had my sons accompany me to my brain-injury support group so they could meet other people who have problems like mine. Unfortunately, the impact of this meeting lasted for only a short time. I often wish that my children would read some of the material available for family members, but it seems their denial and their desire to return to the old days are a stronger force."

—D.R.S.

Denial is the refusal to accept the reality of a problematic condition or event, and it is the biggest obstacle to coping with any injury. In the case of MTBI, where the injury is invisible and the person looks, sounds, and functions (at least in some arenas) as he or she previously did, denial is almost a certainty.

Often, denial starts at the scene of the injury, because police or others in authority make a decision about an individual's need for medical care based upon his or her appearance. You may assume that the injury, if any, must be minor, since the person either was not taken to the hospital at all or was released after superficial examination. If medical help is sought later, the person's complaints are often treated individually—as fatigue or headaches, say—and they may not be linked to the earlier head trauma. If symptoms such as uncharacteristic forgetfulness, poor concentration, irritability, or behavior changes occur, you may first suspect an emotional problem or become impatient when your loved one fails to "snap out of it." Often the injured person, unable to change, becomes depressed.

Realization

If the MTBI person's symptoms persist or intensify, you eventually come to realize that something is wrong and you must give up your denial. With this unwelcome awareness comes fear, worry, and a sense of vulnerability, for you have somehow lost the person you knew and depended upon, and you do not know what the future may bring. Financial issues become a concern, as do home issues such as household responsibilities and the care of children.

Helplessness

"My mother, who has had several strokes, is very understanding, because she has gone through many of the same experiences as I have. However, my extended family has offered limited support because they've done little to educate themselves about my problems. Sometimes I feel like I'm the caregiver and must enlighten everyone, and this is a burden I do not want. I want to feel free to just get better and get on with my life. My saving grace has been psychotherapy, my cyberspace confidantes, and my steadfast friends, who have accepted me and my unpredictability without judgment."

—D.R.S.

If you see someone you care about suffering and behaving in a strange and unpredictable manner, you may feel helpless. Not knowing where to turn or what to do creates an awkwardness that often leads friends and colleagues to stop calling or visiting. Extended family may behave in a similar manner. The immediate family, who cannot practice this kind of avoidance, may instead become withdrawn and extremely impatient.

Frustration

Frustration is an outgrowth of the feelings of helplessness that result from your inability to make things return to normal. There is no question that it can be extremely difficult to deal with an MTBI person's inability to acknowledge his or her deficits and reluctance to make needed lifestyle changes. Often, the injured individual sees his or her primary caregiver as bossy and dominating, and may respond with stubbornness or uncooperativeness, or by giving up household responsibilities. Almost any interaction with the MTBI person can quickly turn into a control issue, leading to anger and conflict in the home.

Anger

Frequently, both the individual with MTBI and his or her family feel anger that the injury has affected their lives. If the trauma was a result of carelessness or some other fault (real or perceived) on the part of the person with MTBI, feelings of anger are intensified. The anger response strains many marriages, and often causes extended family to withdraw emotional support. Friendships that have withstood the stresses so far may fall apart at this point because the friend's anger may not permit him or her to deal with the MTBI person's unpredictability. As a family member or friend, you may feel angry that your loved one has changed so dramatically, often permanently so.

Guilt

Anger at the injured loved one leads to feelings of guilt, as you regret your anger and short-temperedness with someone who badly needs your assistance. You scold yourself for not being more understanding, and feel guilty about not being completely supportive. The fact that you are clearly trying to help does not make you any less ashamed of the annoyance you feel when the MTBI person is being difficult.

Sadness

At some point, perhaps after much time spent going from frustration to anger to guilt and back again, you realize that life with your loved one simply may never be the same. You may get an empty feeling when you look at old photos or when you study the MTBI person as he or she is today. Reminiscing about the past and planning for the future become occasions for feelings of sadness and resignation. There is a genuine loss to be dealt with.

Acceptance

Finally, you learn to accept your injured loved one for who he or she is now. You may not like what has happened to your life, but you accept that your friend or family member, though changed, still has wonderful qualities and many contributions to make to the relationship. You begin to care for and relate to the new person rather than bemoaning the loss of the old. Frustration and anger diminish, and loving interaction returns.

PRACTICAL SUGGESTIONS

"My husband and I have gone to marital counseling to help us cope with my MTBI. I've learned to accept my limitations, lack of reliability, and unpredictability. I've also discovered that it's okay to have someone look out for me. My husband is discovering that my responses aren't always reliable, and that it's not productive to get angry when I do things that he feels are unwise or unsafe."

—D.R.S.

Living with an individual who undergoes the personal changes associated with traumatic brain injury is not easy. It is important to remember that feeling anger or frustration at times is normal, and that despite these feelings, you deserve a great deal of credit for the support and assistance you offer daily. The following are a number of tactics that can help make it easier to deal with a loved one who has had an MTBI:

• Ask your loved one's neurologist about the medical reasons behind the MTBI person's behavioral and other problems. Simply understanding what is really going on may help reduce your frustration.

• Educate yourself about the nature of your friend's or family member's deficits. Refer to the various chapters of this book for hints on coping with specific problems.

• Realize that a person with MTBI passes through several very different phases during recovery. Learn about each stage and try to devise fresh approaches to dealing with it.

• Ask the brain-injured person about how he or she feels, and accept these feelings as real.

• Talk openly about the loss of the "old" person and your frustration with the "new" person's unpredictability.

• Help the injured person set realistic goals and formulate strategies for achieving them. Track your loved one's progress with a success log, and give him or her full credit for everything he or she accomplishes.

• Get to know the new person, and appreciate him or her not in comparison to the old person, but as a valid and worthwhile individual.

• Accept your frustration as normal, but express angry feelings to someone other than the injured person. Find other people in similar situations through support groups and on-line computer services.

- Consider counseling by a professional who specializes in MTBI issues to help you cope with your loved one's difficulties.

- Avoid letting your physical or emotional reserves become drained. Discover what activities refresh and rejuvenate you, and schedule time every week to pursue them. When possible, ask other family members or friends of the person with MTBI to help out.

- Approach memory deficits by taking time to reeducate the person with MTBI about his or her life. For example, look together at old photo albums and family movies and videos.

- Address the person with MTBI by name before asking or telling him or her something important. Doing so increases the chance that your message will be received.

- Focus on the strengths and talents that your loved one still possesses.

- Help your friend or family member learn to live in the outside world again by taking walks together around the yard, neighborhood, and town.

- Find out about services that provide assistance to people with MTBI in the home, workplace, and community. Your local rehabilitation center can advise you as to the types of help that are available.

- Consider personal, couple, or family counseling if coping with your loved one's MTBI is causing emotional or marital problems.

Finally, it is important to realize that you need not be solely in charge of your loved one's recovery. Many types of assistance and support are available to you and the person with MTBI. If you are not sure what type of help you need or where to begin looking, call your state brain-injury association or the national office of the Brain Injury Association for advice and referrals.

Caring for a friend or family member after an MTBI is a huge undertaking, but you need never shoulder the job alone. The ordeal can be lessened by the realization that many postconcussive symptoms lessen with time. As Jeff, whose story opens this chapter, says, "Dealing with a person with MTBI takes patience. . . patience. . . patience."

To Our Caregivers

As we struggle to understand ourselves,
Please understand us too.
As we struggle to learn to accept ourselves,
Accept us too, please do.

As we aspire to reach our goals
Please urge us in that direction.
If we fall short a step or more
Please help us achieve perfection.

Urge us on, but do not push.
Encourage, but do not shove.
We'll be doing our very best
And we will need your love.

The times we are not loveable,
We'll need you all the more!
We'll need you most at the times
When ourselves we do abhor.

And we will promise one thing
Though our progress may be slow;
We'll be doing our very best
As onward we do go.

Onward where? We have no way
Of knowing what the test.
But one thing you can know for sure,
We'll be doing our very best.

—Rita Smithuysen

25

Outcomes of MTBI

Unlike the previous chapters, this chapter does not begin with a real-life story that illustrates a specific problem. This is because each MTBI experience is as unique as the affected individual, and one story alone cannot illustrate the range of outcomes. Since your recovery is unlikely to follow a straight and sure course, your doctor's ability to measure the residual effects of your injury and predict long-term results is limited. Years after suffering an MTBI, some people are fully recovered, while others have learned to accept ongoing symptoms of postconcussive syndrome. Still others may yet be healing, unable to guess at their eventual outcome.

FACTORS THAT INFLUENCE YOUR PROGNOSIS

The outcome of any individual MTBI hinges on the many variables that have been discussed in earlier chapters—among them the site of the injury, the solidity of the person's support system, and the appropriateness of treatment. Your recovery will also be influenced by your preinjury personality and by how determined you are. Age is another factor. Young children and older people, for example, appear to be better able to accept changes in personality and behavior than do young adults. Finances also figure in MTBI outcome. Research has shown that navigating stressful insurance and legal processes related to an accident can hinder recovery. However, while the pace, time frame, and degree of recovery from MTBI may be uncertain, the healing process itself tends to follow a pattern.

The loss of predictability plays a role in recovery from MTBI. Prior to your injury, your life had a certain routine, based in part on your knowledge of how you thought, felt about, and reacted to things. You knew your strengths and weaknesses, what made you angry or sad, and how effective you were on the job. Also, you could plan and organize. Now, no one—including you—may have any idea how you will feel or act at any given time. This loss of predictability is a result of MTBI that may make you feel as if you are always adapting and adjusting your life. Even the experts cannot be certain whether the symptoms of postconcussive syndrome will affect you once a week or once in a lifetime—or, when fatigue, pain, and other maladies do occur, how intense or long-lasting they will be. Therefore, your ability to grieve the loss of who you were before is an extremely important factor in your outcome. Once you let go of the need for predictability and accept your present self, you can once again enjoy life—maybe not as before, but with a new outlook.

STAGES OF RECOVERY

There are several consistent stages in recovery from MTBI. During the first phase, your visible injuries heal enough to make you truly aware of the emotional and cognitive damage left by your MTBI. Often, you notice these changes only when you feel well enough to resume your daily routine and are faced with evidence that you are not the same person as before. As part of this stage of evaluation, you may experience a jumble of feelings, including lack of awareness, denial, anger, depression, and grief. (See Chapters 18 and 21 for more about emotional reactions and grieving the loss of self.)

The second phase of recovery—often the most difficult—has to do with accepting that you may never be the same again. Coping with this realization is made harder each time you catch a glimpse of your "old self" and recognize that some of your former capabilities are out of reach. You live with uncertainty, you struggle to establish new ways of doing things, and you experience setbacks that make you wonder whether you will ever get better. It may be hard to allow others to assist you, but a support system that includes family, friends, and brain-injury support groups is invaluable during the periods of vulnerability and sadness that characterize the second stage of recovery.

As you gradually accept the changes in yourself, you will enter the third phase of healing: regaining independence and a sense of control. You will get a feeling of accomplishment from driving, balancing the checkbook, or recalling a phone number without first writing it down. As you discover that your reactions to situations are quite different than before, you will also learn that there are things about your new personality that you like. You will regain your self-confidence through seemingly minor accomplishments, learn to accept your limitations, and begin to explore previously untapped potential. You will once again make forward progress, although on a different, perhaps bumpier, path than before.

Healing from an MTBI is unlike recovering from an illness. You cannot say at the outset when you will begin to feel better, how you should pass the time, or how much care you would like from others. Instead, you wrestle with unfamiliarity and with friends and family who seem overprotective one minute and pushy the next. But you will achieve a positive outcome when you let go of the "old you," become confident about your new capabilities, and fine-tune the coping skills that allow you to return you to some form of independence.

MTBI OUTCOMES

Throughout this book, you have become acquainted with the thoughts and stories of a number of real individuals as they struggled with the aftermath of MTBI. In this chapter, we will revisit some of these people as they are today, as well as meeting several others who have experienced MTBI. Some of these stories are immensely encouraging, while others may inspire understanding and empathy. Taken together, they serve to illustrate the various and unpredictable courses of recovery from MTBI. You may also recognize elements of your own recovery in these stories.

Beverley's Story

Beverley, the gymnastics judge and real-estate broker whose story was told in Chapters 7 and 12, was in an automobile accident seven years ago and began experiencing complex partial seizures a month afterward. She also completely lost interest in physical intimacy with her husband. Since that time, she has experienced marked improvement. She looks well, her seizures are regulated by medication, and she has completely recovered from her sexual problems. She has written two books, *In Search of Wings* and *To Wherever Oceans Go*; she lectures throughout the United States; and she is active in her family's real-estate firm and is a support counselor at Bayside Rehabilitation in Portland, Maine. Beverley is also the only MTBI survivor who is head of a state head-injury association.

On the flip side, Beverley can never predict how she will be affected by crowds, certain sounds, and crisis situations, or how she will react when crossing a street. During a recent presentation, for example, she needed to have her psychologist sit in the front row for support. When she travels, she always does so with a companion so that she doesn't walk into traffic or misjudge an emergency. But with great determination and a number of life adjustments, Beverley has paved the way to a bright future.

Gracia's Story

Gracia's MTBI, the result of a car accident seven years ago, left her with headaches, dizziness, fatigue, confusion, memory problems, and other mental deficits, as described in the beginning of Chapter 14. Her memory problems improved dramatically after she was taken off several medications for depression. She still has many problems related to organizing, planning, and remembering, but she has devised alternative ways of doing things. For instance, she kept putting freshly made coffee into the garbage. Now she keeps a note on the coffeemaker that says, "Drink it, don't toss it." To avoid the possibility of starting a fire while cooking, Gracia removed the stove from her kitchen and installed a microwave oven.

She is still getting used to the unpredictable new person she has become, but she likes herself more every day. Gracia attributes much of her positive outcome to the unfailing support of her companion and caregiver, Elaine. She also feels that taking care of her pets has forced needed certainty and meaning into her life.

Jack's Story

Jack, the retired law-enforcement officer whose story introduced Chapter 21, still grieves his loss of self from his accident six years ago. He feels he has not yet discovered who he is, because he never knows from moment to moment whether he is going to stutter, feel fatigued, or experience a headache or black mood. He compares his life to an amusement-park ride that takes you into a dark tunnel where you never know what to expect.

Jack has undergone neuropsychological testing and psychotherapy. His participation in a local brain-injury support group has helped him get out of the house and spend time among people who understand him. His clinical depression is being treated with medication, but litigation relating to his accident is pending, and this has caused ongoing stress because he is pressed to report on what he can and cannot do—abilities that vary greatly from day to day. Jack's recovery waxes and wanes, and he senses that he has long road ahead of him.

Mary Beth's Story

Since the skiing accident that caused Mary Beth's MTBI five years ago (described in Chapter 6), she has succeeded both professionally and academically. She is currently a program research specialist at Hudson Valley Community College in New York and teaches three courses there. Her husband, Peter, ultimately found he could not accept that he was living with a new person, and the couple separated. However, Mary Beth's colleagues and close friend Cheryl have been extremely supportive throughout her recovery.

It is Mary Beth's sense of self—of knowing who she is—that has suffered the most. Two years after her injury, she was diagnosed with major depression and placed on medication to help relieve the symptoms, but four months after that, she was nevertheless diagnosed as suicidal. Mary Beth describes herself as having been killed on the mountainside that day five years ago. However, she says she has made many friends through the Internet TBI-Support list and is learning to grieve and go on living with her new, unpredictable self. She calls herself a "functioning dysfunctional."

Jackie's Story

Jackie, a special-education teacher from Minnesota, was a passenger on EgyptAir flight 648 in November of 1985. The plane was hijacked shortly after takeoff, and when it landed for refueling, Jackie was one of a number of passengers who were shot in the head and thrown from the airplane onto the tarmac. Miraculously, she survived. Since that day, needless to say, Jackie's life has totally changed.

In the months following the traumatic event, Jackie suffered from uncontrollable seizures. Her short-term memory was so poor that if she took her eye off an object, it was as if the object never existed. She was also plagued with severe visual and language deficits, mood swings, and flashbacks. As she struggled to cope with these problems, her marriage fell apart.

Jackie's doctors finally found an anticonvulsant that was able to control her seizures, and she sought Gestalt therapy, a form of trauma therapy, to deal with her posttraumatic stress. About 95 percent of her expressive language ability has now returned. Jackie says that if she gets lots of sleep during the night or takes a nap during the day, she can carry on a good conversation. If she is not fatigued, her short-term memory is fairly strong. She still has partial blindness in the top, left, and bottom of her peripheral vision.

Jackie's doctors once told her that with her vision, seizure, and short-term memory problems, she would never go back to work. However, she has proved them wrong. Today, Jackie is the president of her own business and the author of *Miles to Go Before I Sleep*

(Hazelden Publishing, 1996). Her suggestion to other brain-injured people and their families and friends is this: Never give up, always have hope, be patient, and take needed baby steps to get closer to your dreams and goals. Above all else, don't be your own worst enemy. Love who you are—brain injury and all.

Darlene's Story

Darlene, whose story was included in Chapter 10, continues to cook, cater meals for friends, and enter recipe contests using her original recipes. Interestingly, she recently won honorable mention for a recipe she concocted after losing her sense of smell. Today, Darlene's phantom-smell problem is much less troublesome than it was in the months following her MTBI. It comes and goes both without any obvious cause and when triggered by things like a sinus infection or the presence of perfume. In general, Darlene avoids new foods and food products because her missing sense of taste negates their appeal. She worries that in a few years, she will forget what familiar foods taste like.

Darlene says that her husband has been a great help. She asks him whether the house—or she herself—has an odor, and about things like the freshness of foods. She date-labels perishable foods just to be sure. She makes a point of bathing, brushing her teeth, and laundering her clothing quite often so as not to risk odors. For safety, she has a smoke detector and gas alarm in place in her home.

Coping with her sensory problem has taken time, partly because Darlene's doctors initially offered hope that her sense of smell might return, leaving her uncertain as to whether to view her condition as temporary or permanent. Now, she has become resigned to both the loss of smell and taste and her problem with phantom smells.

Mike's Story

Three years ago, Mike was assaulted in his garage by a burglar. He was struck on the head several times and, with the last blow, hit his head on the garage floor. He was left with vision and speech problems that faded after several months.

He still has severe memory loss, however. Mike cannot recall people, places, names, or events, and had to relearn his job among people who were suddenly strangers. He has no memory of his childhood or early adulthood, nor does he remember his parents, children, friends, or even his wedding and honeymoon.

Mike's way of coping is to make new memories, while his wife has become keeper of all that has been important in their past lives. Their loss is painful, but Mike is making progress. His greatest wish is to know his family and friends once again so that life can continue as it was meant to.

Robert's Story

Five years ago, six-year-old Robert was struck on the left side of his head while he and his friends were playing with plastic golf clubs. He seemed fine shortly afterward, but he awoke that night, screaming. An emergency room CT scan showed a subdural hematoma (an accumulation of blood beneath the outermost membrane protecting the brain), and Robert underwent immediate brain surgery.

Robert was left with a number of problems, but most, except for frequent mood swings and short-term memory loss, have improved over time. He was able to begin first grade just a few weeks behind his classmates and by March of the following year, he was attending school full-time. Robert wears a helmet during recess and outdoor contact activities and continues to improve, though he is still frustrated by his changing moods and memory problems. Remarkably, he has accepted that his MTBI changed some of his abilities and that he must retrain himself to learn to compensate for problem areas. He uses cues and visual prompts, for instance, to help him remember things. Robert fully recalls his accident and the events leading up to his surgery, but he has told his mother that the "old" Robert died and there is a "new" Robert recovering.

Laurel's Story

Laurel suffered an MTBI when she sustained a skull fracture and parietal hematoma (an accumulation of blood in the parietal lobe) after a fall from her horse. She underwent emergency surgery to remove the blood clot, and a small section of skull was removed to relieve pressure on her brain. Laurel spent three months at her parents' home recuperating from headaches, dizziness, and short-term memory problems. By the fourth month after her surgery, she was able to return to her work as a physical therapist without any restrictions. Today, Laurel has no residual problems from her injury, and credits her recovery to family support and a strong will to survive.

D.R.S. (My Own Story)

I am still getting used to the new me—a composite of the old and new. I continue to live with physical, emotional, and cognitive problems related to my MTBI, and I can never be sure when I wake up in the morning if I will be able to achieve my goals for the day.

For the first six years after my accident, each day challenged me to find new ways of learning to manage pain, compensate for lost skills, and cope with my emotions and ever-changing symptoms. I used to have an exceptional memory; then it became unpredictable. I could no longer do simple math problems in my head; my judgment was sometimes extremely poor; my mental endurance was compromised to the point that I could not work for more than an hour or two without resting; and I could no longer think and express myself in complicated analogies, but rather had to express myself more simply. Happily, my sexual dysfunction has improved with time and the termination of various medications. There are still some times when I feel absolutely no desire, but this is now the exception rather than the rule.

My fatigue and attention problems affect me the most. For example, my daily activities did not interfere with my work on this book, but I was unable to write new chapters in the presence of my children, a ringing phone, or even my cat entering my office. To prevent myself from losing my thoughts, I need to be able to control my environment. My solution was to isolate myself in a local motel to do my writing.

In the past few years, with the use of the Burdenko method, homeopathics, and psychotherapy, I have made significant progress. My ability to do math has returned, my atypical migraines are under control, and my balance, coordination, and mobility are restored. However, not until six years after my accident, when I discovered the benefits of EEG biofeedback, did my cognitive problems begin to improve markedly. After fifty sessions, I no longer feel fatigue, and my attention, organization skills, and judgment are more consistent. An added bonus was that this treatment eliminated my chronic pain. Now I feel pain only when there is an actual injury to my muscles.

In the years since my MTBI, each day has been a challenge to me. There is no question that my spirit and determination to recover were nurtured by the love of my husband, children, extended family, and close friends. This, along with the care and understanding I received from my local brain-injury support group, friends in the community, and my brain-injured friends on-line, has become the motivating force in my recovery. For instance, when I read what Lianne wrote on a Prodigy MTBI medical support bulletin board about the importance of pets (see page 194), I recalled expressing to my dying cat fears that I never shared with my family or therapist. Another Prodigy writer, Sheila, mentioned that playing the clarinet had helped her. Her words made me reflect upon the healing effect of being once again able to play the guitar. It took me four years, but to my delight, I am able to play again. I sometimes still have problems recalling the lyrics to songs, but I have no difficulty remembering the music.

Sometimes I wish I could take a vacation from myself, but most of the time I am thankful that the new, composite me has the opportunity to meet the challenge of MTBI and watch my children grow up.

YOUR OWN OUTCOME

No one can predict your eventual outcome. Your symptoms may be permanent, come and go unpredictably, or fade altogether. The one factor that can determine your outcome in the way that really counts is you—how you see and accept yourself.

Gail, whose story begins Chapter 4, wrote the following in *The Headliner,* a newsletter of the Oregon Brain Injury Support Group:

> *Our own inner peace will come when we have the strength of mind:*
>
> * *to be satisfied with our own self,*
>
> * *to be accepting of the way we are now,*
>
> * *to be forgiving of ourselves,*
>
> * *to be mindful of our own integrity, and*
>
> * *to let go.*
>
> *Normal? Been there.*
> *Brain damaged? Done that.*
> *Both together? Now there's a real challenge.*

It is my hope that with the information in this book, together with your own acceptance of what you can and cannot do, you can meet this challenge.

CONCLUSION

ON WITH LIVING AGAIN

"Life breaks everyone, but some people become stronger in the broken places."

—*Ernest Hemingway*

You look in the mirror and you appear the same, but you know that a part of you has died. You struggle on a daily basis, wondering why you are no longer reliable, dependable, or predictable. Often, you feel that you are going crazy.

These thoughts and feelings are the same for every person with an MTBI. The purpose of this book has been to help you understand and cope with the residual problems from your brain trauma. You need to know that even if you don't walk, see, or process information the way you once did, you are still a worthwhile person who has much to offer yourself, your family, and society.

It is my hope that this book has provided you with the resources you need to continue your life with dignity and purpose. Use the information to educate yourself about your injury, its aftereffects, and the unpredictability of the healing process. Rely on its chapters to help you select the best treatments and professionals, and to teach the people in your everyday life to help you and listen to you. Ask for help when you are tired, in pain, or unable to do things for yourself. Allow yourself to be emotionally supported by your loved ones, and encourage them to accept you as you are now, rather than focusing on who you were before.

There will be days when your judgment is off, when your memory is unreliable, or when you cannot seem to get past your pain. So too will there be times when you are able to function very well.

Don't forget that before your MTBI, you had good days and bad days, too. Remember that conditions as varied as the barometric pressure, hormonal changes, foods, medication, and the stress of daily living can affect you. Be kind to yourself and use your energy wisely—but don't be afraid to live life. Mourn the loss of the "old you" and enjoy learning all the good things about the "new you." Take a few risks, find humor in everyday things, and reconnect with friends and family at your own pace and on your own level.

The words of the Serenity Prayer provide excellent advice to help you forge through adversity to a new quality of life: Accept the things you cannot change, change the things you can, and try to recognize the difference. Here's wishing you life, and living again!

GLOSSARY

There are many technical terms associated with MTBI and its accompanying symptoms. Understanding these can help you to educate yourself about your problem and work with your physician and other practitioners toward recovery. Some of the most frequently encountered terms are defined below.

absence seizure. A generalized seizure in which consciousness is altered, but without convulsive symptoms. Formerly called *petit mal.*

acalculia. The inability to perform mathematical operations, recognize numbers, or count.

acupuncturist. A practitioner of acupuncture, a type of treatment based on the principles of traditional Chinese medicine, in which extremely fine needles and herbal treatments are used to restore the proper flow of *qi,* or the body's vital energy, to stimulate healing and relieve pain. An acupuncturist must be licensed to provide this service by the state in which he or she practices.

adhesion. A band of fibrous material that forms an abnormal connection between the surface of one internal organ or structure and that of another. Adhesions usually form as a result of scarring.

agitographia. Rapid writing movements with the omission or distortion of letters, words, or parts of words.

agnosia. Loss of comprehension of sensory input, such as sounds or sights. Also, the inability to recognize a familiar object even though all the physical senses are intact and functioning.

agnosia alexia. The inability to comprehend and understand written words.

agraphia. The inability to express thoughts in writing. This can be due to a brain lesion or to muscular coordination problems.

alexia. The inability to read or recognize words.

alexia agraphia. The inability to read and write letters, words, numbers, or musical notes.

amnesia. Loss of memory. *See also* Anterograde amnesia; Retrograde amnesia.

aneurysm. A weak spot in the wall of a blood vessel that may balloon outward and, eventually, rupture. If an aneurysm in a blood vessel in the brain ruptures, brain hemorrhage results.

anomia. An inability to remember names of persons and/or objects.

anosmia. Loss of the sense of smell.

anoxia. Lack of oxygen. Anoxia in brain tissue causes brain injury.

anterior. Pertaining to the front part of a structure.

anterograde amnesia. Inability to remember a traumatic event, such as a brain injury, and events that occurred afterward. Also called *posttraumatic amnesia.*

anticonvulsant. Medication used to prevent seizures by suppressing irregular electrical discharges in the brain.

aphasia. An inability to express coherent ideas or understand spoken language. *See also* Conductive aphasia; Expressive aphasia; Receptive aphasia.

apraxia. Difficulty starting, continuing, and stopping movements even though there is no actual muscle weakness, paralysis, or sensory change or damage. Apraxia may affect speech or the movement of the arms and legs. Also called motor planning problems.

articulation. The ability to correctly pronounce the speech sounds in words.

astereognosis. The inability to recognize objects or shapes by feeling them.

ataxia. An inability to coordinate muscle movements and action that is not due to apraxia (see above), to the extent that the ability to walk, talk, eat, work, and perform self-care tasks is compromised.

attention. The ability to focus on specific messages for a period of time while screening out irrelevant information.

audiologist. A professional who assesses hearing deficits through the interpretation of an audiogram, or hearing test.

aura. An early neurlogical symptom that may precede a migraine or a seizure. An aura may manifest itself as bodily sensations, sounds, smells, visual images, flashing lights, the sudden development of a blind spot, and/or a feeling of spaciness.

behavior. The total collection of overt actions and reactions exhibited by a person.

behavioral neurologist. A medical doctor who is a specialist in neurology and the treatment of organic personality change.

biofeedback. A technique utilizing an external monitoring system to help an individual become conscious of usually unconscious body processes, such as the activities of the muscular, thermal, and electrical systems of the body. This makes it possible to gain some measure of conscious control over these processes, and thereby learn to manage headaches, chronic pain, and other problems.

brain plasticity. The ability of noninjured brain cells to take over functions of damaged cells.

brain stem. The rear lower part of the brain, just above the spinal cord. It contains the midbrain, the pons, and the medulla oblongata, structures that control breathing and heartbeat, and serves as a relay station for all motion and sensation.

central nervous system (CNS). The part of the nervous system made up of the brain and spinal cord.

cerebellum. The portion of the brain that is located below the cerebrum and is concerned with coordinating movements. Damage to this area may result in ataxia.

cerebral cortex. *See* Cerebrum.

cerebrospinal fluid (CSF). A colorless solution of sodium chloride and other salts that circulates around the brain and spinal cord.

cerebrum. The largest and most advanced part of the brain. It consists of two hemispheres connected by a band of tissue. It is the area where most cognitive functions (thinking, understanding, and reasoning) take place. It is divided into four lobes: the frontal, temporal, parietal, and occipital. Also called the *cortex* or *cerebral cortex.*

chiropractor. A practitioner of chiropractic, a hands-on technique of manipulating the spine and/or joints to promote healing and relieve pain. A chiropractor must be licensed by the state in which he or she practices.

circumlocution. Talking around an idea without ever coming to the point.

clinical social worker. A social worker who specializes in emotional and mental disorders. Many clinical social workers provide psychotherapy services.

CNS. *See* central nervous system (CNS).

cognition. The process of thinking, understanding, and reasoning.

cognitive flexibility. The ability to shift from one task to another.

coma. An unconscious state that lasts longer than an hour.

complex partial seizure. A seizure that involves only part of the brain—usually the frontal or temporal lobe—and causes an alteration of consciousness.

comprehension. The ability to understand things that are heard, seen, and/or touched.

computed tomography scan (CT scan). A diagnostic test that uses x-rays and computer analysis to produce a picture of the brain.

concentration. The capacity to maintain undivided attention on a specific message or task.

concussion. A blow to the head that causes unconsciousness but no observable disruption of nerve impulses in the brain. Also called *diffuse traumatic brain injury.*

conductive aphasia. A language problem characterized by halting speech with word-finding pauses and repetition of words.

confabulation. An attempt to compensate for memory loss by making things up to fill in and cover up gaps in memory.

consulting physician. A physician contacted by a primary health-care provider for professional advice about specific aspects of a patient's care.

contusion. An injury that results in localized bruising, swelling, and hemorrhaging from capillaries. A contusion in the brain can result in MTBI.

convulsion. Involuntary, spasmodic, usually full-body muscle contractions. At one time, the word *convulsion* was used interchangeably with *seizure*, but this is no longer the case.

corpus callosum. The band of nerve fibers that connects the right and left hemispheres of the brain and allows for rapid and effective communication between hemispheres.

cortex. *See* Cerebrum.

cortical blindness. Severe loss of vision in both eyes caused by damage to the vision nerves in the brain's occipital lobe.

coup/contrecoup. Literally, "blow/counterblow." A type of head injury in which impact on one place on the head causes the brain to bounce against the opposite side of the skull, thereby causing injury to both sides of the brain.

CSF. *See* cerebrospinal fluid (CSF).

CT scan. *See* Computed tomography scan.

déjà vu. A sense that you have seen, done, or experienced something before, whether or not you actually have. In a person with MTBI, this can occur because of a total lack of awareness that he or she is recalling past information.

denial. The failure or refusal to accept the reality of something, such as brain injury.

diffuse brain damage. Damage affecting many areas of the brain rather than one specific location.

diplopia. Double vision; perception of two images from a single object.

disinhibition. Loss of restraint; a decrease in the ability to stop oneself from saying or doing things that are typically inappropriate or undesirable.

disorientation. A disturbance in the recognition of people, places, and/or time and day; not knowing where you are or who you are.

dysarthria. Problems with the muscle movements needed to form, or articulate, words. Dysarthria affects the pronounation of spoken sounds.

dyscalculia. Partial inability to perform mathematical functions.

dysfluency. Stuttering; repetition or drawing out of initial word sounds.

dysgraphia. Partial inability to perform the motor movements required for writing.

dyslexia. A partial inability to read words, characterized by misperception of letters and letter sequences, misidentification of words, and/or an inability to distinguish text from its background.

dysnomia. Difficulty finding and retrieving words.

dysosmia. An altered sense of smell.

dyspraxia. A partial loss of the ability to perform skilled, coordinated movements even though there is no defect in motor or sensory function.

dyssymbolia. A partial loss of the ability to use or understand symbols, such as those used in mathematics, chemistry, or music.

EEG. *See* electroencephalogram.

electroencephalogram (EEG). A diagnostic test that records electrical activity in the brain.

emotional lability. Intense fluctuations of emotion that appear to be exaggeraged or inappropriate responses to situations or thoughts, or that occur without any reason.

epilepsy. A disorder characterized by recurring seizures.

expressive aphasia. A problem with expressive language, such as difficulty in articulation, fluency, and written communication. Also called *Broca's aphasia.*

factitious disorder. The intentional falsification of illness by pretending or inflicting injury on oneself, even though one does not stand to gain anything by doing so.

fascia. A covering over a muscle that allows it to glide over adjacent muscle.

floaters. Tiny bits of solid matter that develop in the vitreous fluid, the gel-like substance that fills most of the space within the back half of the space within the eyeball, between the lens and the retina, causing one to see tiny floating spots.

frontal lobe. The area of the brain located at the front, closest to the forehead. It is responsible for emotions, behaviors, social and motor skills, abstract thinking, reasoning, planning, judgment, and memory.

gustatory. Pertaining to the sense of taste.

hematoma. An accumulation of escaped blood trapped within an organ or tissue, usually the result of injury.

hemiparesis. Weakness of one side or part of the body due to injury to motor areas of the brain.

hemiplegia. Paralysis of one side of the body.

hemorrhage. Abnormal discharge of blood.

herbalist. A practitioner who prescribes various types of herbal remedies to stimulate healing and harmony within the body.

homeopath. A practitioner who treats illness by prescribing homeopathic remedies, which consist of highly diluted plant, animal, and mineral substances. Remedies are prescribed based on a detailed, multifaceted evaluation of symptoms.

hyposmia. A partial loss of the sense of smell.

hypothalamus. The part of the brain that influences sex drive, sleep, body temperature, appetite, long-term memory, and the expression of emotion.

hypotonicity. Abnormally low muscle tone, primarily in the trunk but also in the extremities.

IBS. *See* Interictal behavior syndrome.

ice-pick headache. A sudden, brief, severe stabbing pain on the surface of the head.

ictal event. A medical term for a seizure of any type.

ictus. Latin for "event." A seizure may be referred to as an ictus. *See also* Ictal event.

initiation. In behavioral terms, the ability to carry out tasks you have set for yourself.

interictal behavior syndrome (IBS). A long-term, dramatic personality difference exhibited by some seizure sufferers. The syndrome is often characterized by biological changes such as depression, diminished sexuality, or increased aggression. An affected individual may also become preoccupied with mystical thinking or feelings of extrasensory perception, or become unusually wordy and obsessed with details.

judgment. The ability to make appropriate decisions based on information and possible consequences.

laterality. The property of relating to one side of the body or the other.

lesion. A visible localized abnormality of the tissues of the body; any damage to the nervous system.

limbic system. A group of interconnected deep-brain structures that helps the hypothalamus prioritize incoming information and also plays a part in controlling memory and emotion.

magnetic resonance imaging (MRI). An imaging test that uses a magnetic field and a computer to produce an image of the brain or other internal structures; it produces a clearer picture than x-rays or a CT scan.

malingering. The intentional falsification of illness by pretending or inflicting injury on oneself in order to gain financial compensation or avoid work, military duty, or criminal prosecution.

memory. A complex process of storing and retrieving information for later use. Types of memory include sensory/immediate, or information that lasts for a second; short-term/working, or information that lasts up to one minute; and long-term/secondary, or information that lasts longer than one minute.

Ménière's syndrome. A condition characterized by one-sided low-frequency hearing loss with a sensation of fullness in the same ear; ringing or buzzing noises in the ear; and severe, even violent, attacks of vertigo.

meninges. Any one of three membranes—the dura mater, pia mater, and the arachnoid—that enclose the brain and spinal cord.

migraine. A neurological disorder caused by blood-vessel or electrical-impulse changes in the brain and characterized by intense headache, often affecting only one side of the head, that may be preceded by an aura and/or accompanied by nausea, vomiting, and/or sensitivity to light and noise. In some cases, symptoms can be almost identical to those of a seizure. A migraine preceded by an aura is termed a *classic migraine* or *migraine with aura*; a migraine not preceded by an aura is called a *common migraine* or *migraine without aura*.

motor planning problems. *See* Apraxia.

MRI. *See* magnetic resonance imaging.

muscular therapist. A specialist who uses therapeutic muscular massage to treat a variety of conditions and complaints.

neurologist. A medical doctor who specializes in the nervous system and its disorders.

neuropsychologist. A psychologist with special training in the relationship between behavior and the brain. Neuropsychologists assess problems with brain function and coordinate the rehabilitation of brain-behavior relationships.

nystagmus. Involuntary horizontal, vertical, or rotary movement of the eyeball.

occipital lobe. The posterior, or back, part of the brain. This area is involved in perceiving and understanding visual information.

occupational therapist. A specialist in upper-extremity rehabilitation. Occupational therapy improves the fine motor, social, and daily living skills of people challenged by a brain or bodily injury, and teaches people how to contribute to their own recovery and avoid reinjury.

olfactory. Pertaining to the sense of smell.

ophthalmologist. A medical doctor who specializes in the diagnosis and medical and surgical treatment of eye disorders.

optometrist. A practitioner who evaluates vision and prescribes corrective lenses, and provides testing for certain eye disorders. An optometrist must be licensed by the state in which he or she practices.

orientation. Awareness of self in relation to person, place, and time, in past or present environments.

orthopedist. A medical doctor who specializes in the musculoskeletal system and its disorders.

otolaryngologist. A medical doctor with expertise in the field of ear and hearing disorders; an ear/nose/throat (ENT) specialist.

paraphasia. A speech problem characterized by the substitution of parts or syllables of words for the actual words.

parietal lobe. The upper middle section of the brain. This area is responsible for sensory and spatial awareness, giving feedback from and understanding of eye, hand, and arm movements during complex operations such as reading, writing, and numerical calculations.

peripheral nerves. Nerves that lie outside the brain and spinal cord.

perseveration. Uncontrollable repetition of speech or movement.

phonophobia. Abnormal sensitivity to noise. Phonophobia is often experienced during a migraine attack.

photophobia. Abnormal sensitivity to light. Photophobia is often experienced during a migraine attack.

physiatrist. A medical doctor who specializes in physical medicine and rehabilitation. Pronounced fizz-EYE-a-trist.

physical therapist. A therapist trained in muscle rehabilitation. Physical therapists use a variety of techniques, including massage, water therapy, hot packs, ice massage, ultrasound, and therapeutic exercises to reduce pain and help patients improve or regain physical functioning.

polarity therapist. A practitioner who uses therapeutic touch and relaxation techniques to promote bodily harmony and healing.

pons. A prominence in the brain stem located between the medulla oblongata and the midbrain.

posterior. Pertaining to the back part of a structure.

posttraumatic amnesia. *See* Anterograde amnesia.

posttraumatic headache. A type of headache that results from a head injury, sometimes persisting for a year or longer after the trauma.

premorbid. Prior to injury or the onset of illness.

primary health-care provider. A family physician, general practitioner, homeopathic physician, or other practitioner who sees to a person's routine health-care needs and provides referrals to specialists for evaluation of certain medical problems.

prognosis. A forecast as to the likely outcome of an illness or injury.

prosopagnosia. The inability to recognize faces.

psychiatric nurse clinical specialist. A nurse with a master's degree in psychiatric mental health nursing who can prescribe and administer medication with special certification. He or she has expertise in medical issues and the diagnosis, treatment, and prevention of emotional and mental disorders.

psychiatrist. A medical doctor licensed to prescribe medication who has expertise in the diagnosis, treatment, and prevention of emotional, behavioral, and mental disorders.

psychologist. A doctor of psychology who is licensed to assess, diagnose, and treat emotional and mental disorders and who oversees the management of attitude and behavioral problems. Psychologists do not prescribe medication. Many psychologists hold board certification in specialty areas of psychology, such as behavioral medicine.

psychopharmacologist. A medical doctor who is a specialist in psychiatry and has expertise in the use and interactions of medication to treat neurological, psychological, and behavioral problems.

quadriparesis. A weakness that involves all four limbs.

receptive aphasia. A term that denotes problems with reading, interpreting, and comprehending spoken language. Also called *Wernicke's aphasia,* this problem affects the ability to understand the meaning of spoken and written words.

rehabilitation. A program or process designed to reduce deficits following injury or illness, and to assist a person in attaining his or her optimal level of mental and physical functioning. Rehabilitation may involve working on an outpatient basis with one or more specialists. Pain management techniques may also be involved.

retrograde amnesia. Inability to recall events prior to a traumatic event. The "missing" memories may cover a specific span of time or certain information.

seizure. A sudden, temporary, unusual discharge of electrical impulses within one area of the brain that may quickly spread to other areas, causing uncontrolled stimulation of nerves and muscles. Seizures usually last only a few minutes and can cause abnormal or arrested movement, alteration of consciousness, disorders of sensation or perception, and behavior disturbances. Also called an *ictal event.*

sequelae. The consequences that follow an illness or injury.

shearing. A type of brain lesion often seen as a result of an abrupt deceleration in movement that causes the brain to continue moving within the skull, tearing brain cells.

somatoform disorder. The presence of one or more physical complaints for which a physical explanation cannot be found.

somatogenic. A disorder or disease with clear-cut physical origins.

sound agnosia. The inability to understand environmental sounds, such as the barking of a dog, without an accompanying disturbance in the ability to understand speech.

spasticity. A condition of spasms or other uncontrollable contractions of the skeletal muscles.

speech/language therapist or pathologist. A practitioner who specializes in the evaluation of speech and language deficits and devises individualized therapy programs consisting of tasks and exercises to improve concentration, articulation, and listening and comprehension skills.

stereognosis. The inability to recognize objects by the sense of touch.

strephosymbolia. The perception of words in reverse or twisted order.

syncope. Medical term for a fainting episode, characterized by dizziness and sweating followed by a loss of consciousness.

syndrome. Not a disease, but a collection of signs or symptoms that together form a condition that has a known outcome or that requires special treatment.

temporal lobe. A part of the brain located beneath the frontal and parietal lobes that plays a part in remembering information, noticing things, understanding music, categorizing objects, the ability to smell and taste, and sexual and aggressive behavior. At the back of the left temporal lobe is *Wernicke's area,* which is responsible for hearing and interpreting language.

tension headache. A two-sided headache caused by muscle tension that feels like squeezing or pressure of a tight band around your head. It may be accompanied by facial or back pain, particularly in persons who have had a whiplash injury.

thalamus. Part of the brain that acts as a nerve-impulse relay station for information being sent to and from the brain, passing it to the *hypothalamus* to be screened and transmitted throughout the body.

thunderclap headache. A sudden, excruciating headache that may reflect bleeding into the head.

tinnitus. A condition characterized by persistent roaring, buzzing, or ringing in the ears.

tone. The tension in resting muscles and the amount of resistance felt when a muscle is moved.

topographagnosia. Problems with route-finding or the understanding or reading of maps.

tracking. The ability to maintain visual focus on a moving object.

tremor. Rhythmic, purposeless, quivering movements resulting from the involuntary contraction and relaxation of opposing groups of muscles.

verbal apraxia. Impaired control of the sequencing of muscles used in speech; specifically, the tongue, lips, jaw muscles, and vocal cords. These muscles are not weak but their control is defective, causing speech to be labored and characterized by sound reversals, additions, and word approximations.

vestibular stimulation. A type of treatment in which movement is used to stimulate the balance mechanism of the inner ear.

visual agnosia. Partial or complete inability to understand things that are seen, even though the sense of sight is functioning normally.

visual-field deficit. An inability to see something in a specific area of the visual field. Often, either the left or right half of the field of vision is involved.

visual-spatial agnosia. Problems with understanding external environmental relationships.

RESOURCES

Listed below are sources of assistance with and information concerning MTBI, including medical treatment, educational information, and referrals to different types of health-care providers, as well as legal assistance and rehabilitation services. Be aware that addresses and telephone numbers are subject to change.

In addition to organizations and individual people, this list includes on-line services that provide support, encouragement, and other types of assistance beneficial to brain-injured persons. There is much health-related information available on-line. Here too, you should be aware that addresses are subject to change. Also, new resources are appearing all the time. In addition to consulting the sites listed in this section, you may wish to search for others on your own. To search for additional sites, you must first be connected to the Internet through an on-line service provider, then connect to a search engine. Search engines are websites that enable you to locate other places on the Internet that pertain to a given topic. When the search engine site comes up on your screen, you enter a few keywords or navigate through a series of indices to find links to sites on that topic. Some search engines you may find useful include the following: Alta Vista (http://altavista.digital.com); Excite (http://www.excite.com); Hotbot (http://www.hotbot.com); Infoseek (http://guide.infoseek.com); Lycos (http://www.lycos.com); Magellan (http://www.mckinley.com); Open Text (http://index.opentext.net); Web Crawler (http://webcrawler.com); and Yahoo (http://www.yahoo.com). There are also a number of specifically medically-oriented search engines. These include: Achoo (http://www.achoo.com) and HealthAtoZ (http://www.Healthatoz.com).

BRAIN INJURY

Organizations

Brain Injury Association (BIA)
1776 Massachusetts Avenue NW, Suite 100
Washington, DC 20036
Telephone: (202) 296–6443
Family hotline: (800) 444–6443
Website: http://www.biausa.org

This organization provides information, publications, and referrals to local chapters in support of brain-injured people, their families, and medical professionals, as well as referrals to rehabilitation centers that provide compensatory memory training and assistance in securing counseling and other services. Referrals are also made to other state and local brain-injury organizations. You can obtain a catalogue of educational materials that cover, in addition to general information on TBI, such topics as youth and TBI; adults and TBI; research; family issues; substance abuse; legal issues; economic issues; advocacy; choosing services; and treatment and rehabilitation issues.

The Perspectives Network
P.O. Box 1859
Cumming, GA 30128-1859
Telephone: (334) 639–5037, (800) 685–6302 (USA only)
Fax (770) 844–6898
E-mail:dtaylor@tbi.org
Website: http://www.tbi.org

This international nonprofit organization was founded in 1990 by a survivor of acquired brain injury. TPN offers a monthly publication and on-line resource information and support dealing with the consequences of traumatic brain injury. For a list of publications, send a self-addressed legal-size envelope with seventy-eight cents postage.

Websites

Centre for Neuro Skills—TBI Resource Guide
http://www.callamer.com/~cns/

This site provides links to information about CNS, rehabilitation, neurolinks, and a brain glossary.

Domestic Engineer Network
http://www.geocities.com/Heartland/Hill/1876

This website was designed by a TBI person named Rose. The purpose is to provide a site where people can exchange thoughts, poetry, humor, and general information.

Head Injury: A NARIC Resource Guide for People With Head Injuries
   and Their Families
http://www.cais.net/naric/hi.html

This guide contains educational information and provides a resource list of a variety of telephone hotlines, magazines, newsletters, pamphlets, and books. It also provides links to other TBI sites.

rehabNet
http://rehabnet.com

This is the website of the Northeast Rehabilitation Hospital in Salem, New Hampshire. It contains articles on ABI/TBI, along with information about this hospital's services.

TBI Chat
http://www.tbi.org/html/chat.html

On this web page, there are links to the Brain Injury Association and many of the individual websites of state brain-injury associations; a brain map; the veterans' head-injury program; the encephalitis support group; and a link to brain-injury groups by state.

The ABI/TBI Information Project
http://www.sasquatch.com/tbi/

This site provides e-mail information, articles, TBI support material, and information on how to subscribe to TBI support newsgroups.

The Neurotrauma Law Nexus
http://www.neurolaw.com

This site provides information about incidence, causes, and consequences of TBI. It is a link to many useful resources.

On-Line Services

Prodigy

Prodigy has a brain-injury bulletin-board service and chat area (you must be a Prodigy subscriber to access these services).
   Chat area: Go to Chat, then select Medical Health 1, Brain Injury

Support. Hours are 3:00 P.M. Eastern time Tuesday and 9:00 P.M. Eastern time Friday. For more information, send e-mail to Bryttel (the chat session moderator) at ZQQM60E@prodigy.com.

Bulletin board: Go to /Jump: Medical support BB. Select topic: Neurological. Select subject: Brain Injury-Coping.

TBI Newsgroup
bit.listserv.tbi-support

Also called Usenet or Netnews, this resembles a global bulletin-board system. Each item that someone posts is passed from system to system. This newsgroup can be found through any of the on-line services, Netscape, and Internet Explorer. You can freely read the messages, but must subscribe to the area if you wish to post messages. To subscribe, send e-mail to listserv@maelstrom.stjohns.edu. Leave the subject line blank. In the body of the message, write subscribe tbi-sprt.

In addition to the above, America Online (AOL), the Microsoft Network (MSN), and CompuServe all have some type of bulletin-board service available to post messages to someone with a TBI; however, none has a chat area specifically for TBI.

AOL: Message board—Better Health Medical Forum, TBI.
CompuServe: Message board (Go Goodhealth); Folder: TBI.
MSN: Post messages.

OTHER HEALTH ISSUES

Organizations

American Academy of Ophthalmology
655 Beach Street
San Francisco, CA 94109-1336
Telephone: (415) 561–8500
Website: http://www.eyenet.org

This association of ophthalmologists conducts research into diseases and treatment of the eye, establishes eye-care policies, and furnishes educational pamphlets and local referrals. Its website has graphics depicting eye anatomy and information on conditions and treatment.

American Academy of Otolaryngology—Head and Neck Surgery
1 Prince Street
Alexandria, VA 22314
Telephone: (703) 836–4444

Website: http://www.entnet.org
This organization of otolaryngologists undertakes research into disorders of the ear, nose, and throat; provides local referrals; and publishes brochures and other public service materials.

American Chronic Pain Association
P.O. Box 850
Rocklin, CA 95677
Telephone: (916) 632–0922
E-mail: acpa@pacbell.net

This organization dispenses information about coping with pain and furnishes referrals to over 800 affiliated pain-management support groups.

American Council for Headache Education (ACHE)
875 Kings Highway, Suite 200
Woodbury, NJ 08096-3172
Telephone: (609) 845–0322 (in New Jersey),
    (800) 255–ACHE (elsewhere)
Fax: (609) 384–5811
E-mail: headquarters@ache.ccmail.compuserve.com
Website: http://www.achenet.org

This nonprofit organization is dedicated to public education, scientific research, and advocacy for people who experience headaches. ACHE also sponsors a number of on-line outlets, including a message board, monthly conference, and chat area on CompuServe; a message board and chat session on America On-line; and a bulletin board and chat session on Prodigy. These can be found as follows:
CompuServe
    Chat area: Health & Fitness Forum, Headache/Migraine conference room R2. Hours are 9:00–10:00 P.M. Eastern time every Sunday.
    Message Board (Go Goodhealth).
America Online
    Headache Chat: Private room "Haches." Days and times posted on message board.
    Message Board: Better Health Medical Forum.
Prodigy
    Bulletin Board: Medical Support, Migraine, Headache (MHA).
    Chat session times: 9:00–10:00 P.M. Eastern time every Thursday.

American Hearing Research Foundation
55 East Washington Street, Suite 2022
Chicago, IL 60602
Telephone: (312) 726–9670
Fax: (312) 726–9695

This association supports research and education concerning hearing disorders, and offers a newsletter and semiannual progress report regarding developments in the field.

American Medical Association (AMA)
515 North State Street
Chicago, IL 60610
Telephone: (312) 464–5000
http://www.ama-assn.org/

This member organization for physicians offers various publications and educational services, and has a consumer book department.

American Pain Society
4700 West Lake Avenue
Glenview, IL 60025
Telephone: (847) 375–4715
E-mail: aps@amctec.com
Website: http://www.ampainsoc.org

This division of the American Academy of Pain Medicine offers information and referrals to people suffering chronic pain.

American Psychiatric Association
1400 K Street, NW
Washington, DC 20005
Telephone: (202) 682–6000
E-mail: apa@psych.org
Website: http://www.psych.org

This scientific and professional society provides scientific and educational resources and referrals for psychiatrists and psychopharmacologists in your locality.

American Psychological Association
750 First Street, NE
Washington, DC 20006-4242
Telephone: (202) 336–5500
E-mail: helping@apa.org
Website: http://www.apa.org

This professional society provides scientific and educational resources and referrals for clinical psychologists, health psychologists, and neuropsychologists in specific localities.

American Speech-Language, Hearing Association
10801 Rockville Pike
Rockville, MD 20852
Telephone: (800) 498–2071 or (301) 897–8682
TTY: (301) 897–8682
Website: http://www.asha.org

This nonprofit organization provides educational information on speech, language, and hearing disabilities. The association publishes pamphlets and other literature on a wide range of communication disorders. It also provides referrals for speech and language pathologists in specific localities.

American Tinnitus Association
P.O. Box 5
Portland, OR 98207
Telephone: (503) 248–9985
E-mail: tinnitus@ata.org
Website: http://www.teleport.com/~ata

This group furnishes information about tinnitus and provides referrals to local support groups and doctors who specialize in treating the condition.

Association for Research in Vision and Ophthalmology
9650 Rockville Pike
Bethesda, MD 20814-3998
Telephone: (301) 571–1844
E-mail: admin@arvo.arvo.org
Website: http://www.arvo.org/arvo/.

This organization of eye care professionals encourages research into eye disorders and offers publications as well as referrals to local eye-care services.

Better Hearing Institute
P.O. Box 1840
Washington, DC 20013
Telephone: (703) 642–0580
E-mail: betterhearing@juno.com
Website: http://www.betterhearing.org

This organization seeks to inform the public about the nature of hearing loss and the various medical, surgical, rehabilitative, and amplification techniques that are available.

Epilepsy Foundation of America
4351 Garden City Drive
Landover, MD 20785
Telephone: (800) 332–1000
Website: http://www.efa.org

This organization supports medical, social, rehabilitative, legal, employment, and informational programs that assist people with seizure disorders. The foundation sponsors research, publishes educational materials, and provides information, referrals, and many types of support.

Epilepsy Services of Southeast Florida
5730 Corporate Way, Suite 220
West Palm Beach, FL 33407-2032
Telephone: (561) 478–6515
E-mail: epilepsy@maco.net
Website: http://seflin.lib.fl.us/epilepsy/index.html

This organization helps people affected by seizures. Programs and services include medical and seizure-control clinic, early recognition and response, support groups, prevention and educational information, and summer camp.

Grief Recovery Helpline
Telephone: (800) 445–4808

This nonprofit organization of staff and volunteers helps people to deal with grief.

House Ear Institute
2100 West 3rd Street, 5th Floor
Los Angeles, CA 90057
Telephone: (213) 483–4431
Website: http://www.hei.org

This professional group develops approaches to hearing and balance disorders through applied research. The institute maintains a library and publishes a number of educational materials.

Learning Disabilities Association of America (LDA)
4156 Library Road
Pittsburgh, PA 15234
Telephone: (412) 341–1515
E-mail: ldanatl@usaor.net
Website: http://www.ldanatl.org

This organization seeks to advance the education and well-being of children

*with learning disabilities by providing information and supporting research
and related services.*

Ménière's Network
Ear Foundation
1817 Patterson
Nashville, TN 37203
Telephone: (615) 329–7807
E-mail: EARFYI@aol.com
Website: http://www.theearfound.com

*This support organization offers help to people with Ménière's syndrome in
the form of educational programs and materials. The group also maintains a
speakers' bureau.*

National Center for Learning Disabilities (NCLD)
381 Park Avenue South, Suite 1420
New York, NY 10016
Telephone: (212) 545–7510
Website: http://www.ncld.org

*This nonprofit organization develops programs and seminars dealing with
learning disabilities, offers resources and referrals to remedial specialists, and
takes part in legislative advocacy and public-awareness campaigns.*

National Eye Institute
NIH, Building 31, Room 6A32
Bethesda, MD 20892-2510
Telephone: (301) 496–5248
E-mail: 2020@b31.nei.nih.gov
Website: http://www.nei.nih.gov

*This division of the National Institutes of Health runs the National Eye
Health Education Program and publishes pamphlets and other educational materials about treatment of eye disorders.*

National Eye Research Foundation
910 Skokie Boulevard, Suite 207A
Northbrook, IL 60062
Telephone: (847) 564–4652
E-mail: nerf1955@aol.com
Website: http://www.eyemac.com/NERF

*This group of eye-care professionals sponsors research into and education about
eye care. The organization serves as a public information center for questions
about the eyes, maintains a library, and offers various publications.*

National Institute of Deafness and Other Communication Disorders
(NIDCD)
Information Clearinghouse
1 Communication Avenue
Bethesda, MD 20892-3456
Telephone: (800) 241–1044
TTY: (800) 241–1055
E-mail: nidcd@aerie.com
Website: http://www.nih.gov/nidcd/

*This institute funds research in taste and smell disorders. The clearinghouse
provides information about hearing, balance, smell and taste, voice, and speech
and language, as well as referrals to NIDCD-funded research and training
centers.*

National Institute of Neurological Disorders and Stroke
Building #31, Room 8A06
31 Center Drive
Bethesda, MD 20892-2540
Telephone: (301) 496–5751
Website: http://www.ninds.nih.gov

*This government organization provides educational material and information
about neurological conditions.*

The People's Pharmacy
P.O. Box 52027
Durham, NC 27717

*This organization dispenses advice and information concerning medication, and
offers a booklet about sexual side effects and alternatives called* Graedon's
Guide to Drugs that Affect Sexuality. *Mail inquiries only.*

Recovery of Male Potency
27211 Lasher Road, Suite 202
Southfield, MI 48034
Telephone: (810) 357–1314

This local support organization offers information and educational material.

Speak Easy International Foundation
233 Concord Drive
Paramus, NJ 07652
Telephone: (201) 262–0895

This support organization and information source serves individuals with speech disorders. The group seeks to instill confidence, reinforce fluency, and educate the public, families, and friends about the problems faced by dysfluent individuals.

The Simon Foundation for Continence
P.O. Box 835
Wilmette, IL 60091
Telephone: (800) 237–4666
E-mail: robmark@integrated-marketing.com
Website: http://www.tbilaw.com

This nonprofit organization provides informational material along with numerous links to other TBI sites.

University of Connecticut
Connecticut Chemosensory Clinical Research Center
263 Farmington Avenue
Farmington, CT 06030-5385
Telephone: (860) 679–2459
E-mail: amot@neuron.uchc.edu
Website: http://www3.uchc.edu/~taste

The clinic evaluates and manages patients with disorders of taste and smell and burning-mouth problems.

Vestibular Disorders Association
P.O. Box 4467
Portland, OR 97208-4467
Telephone: (503) 229–7705
Fax: (503) 229–8064
E-mail: veda@teleport.com
Website: http://www.teleport.com/~veda

This organization offers support services and referrals to people suffering from vestibular problems. The association maintains a library and encourages public education through booklets and newsletters.

Websites

MedicineNet
http://www.medicinenet.com

The content of this site includes interactive groups, ask-the-doctor features, a medical dictionary, comprehensive drug information, medical news, disease-specific information, and links to other sites.

GlobalMedic
http://www.globalmedic.com

This site is an encyclopedia of medical terms, with special sections for women and children.

Global Navigator Alternative Medicine Site
http, http://www.arxc.com

This is a general site about alternative medicine. It has links to other sites.

Internet Mental Health Home Page
http://www.mentalhealth.com/

This site provides information about mental health and links to other sites.

Medscape
http://www.medscape.com

This site has the full text of articles from such sources as the National Institutes of Health and the Centers for Disease Control and Prevention.

The University of Pittsburgh Alternative Medicine Home Page
http://www.pitt.edu/~cbw/altm.html

This site provides general inforamtion about alternative medicine and links to other sites.

Yahoo-Health:Medicine:Neurosciences
http://www.yahoo.com/health/medicine/neurosciences

This site provides links to major TBI and other sites.

TREATMENT APPROACHES

Organizations

Alternative Therapies in Health and Medicine
Innovision Communication
101 Columbia Aliso
Viejo, CA 92656
Telephone: (714) 362–2000, (800) 899–1712
E-mail: alttherapy@aol.com
Website: http://www.healthonline.com/altther.htm

Alternative Therapies is a forum for sharing information concerning the practical use of alternative therapies in preventing and treating disease, healing illness, and promoting health.

American Association of Oriental Medicine
433 Front Street
Catasauqua, PA 18032
Telephone: (610) 266–1433
Fax: (610) 264–2768
E-mail: aaom1@aol.com
Website: http://www.aaom.org

This nonprofit organization provides educational materials and referrals to acupuncturists in specific localities.

American Association of Sex Educators, Counselors, and Therapists
P.O. Box 238
Mt. Vernon, IA 52314-0238
Telephone: (319) 895–8407

This professional organization offers educational information and referrals, and publishes comprehensive directories of certified specialists.

American Chiropractic Association (ACA)
1701 Clarendon Boulevard
Arlington, VA 22209
Telephone: (703) 276–8800
E-mail: acamic@erols.com
Website: http://www.amerchiro.org

This professional organization provides educational information and referrals to practitioners in specific localities.

American Dance Therapy Association (ADTA)
2000 Century Plaza, Suite 108
10632 Little Patuxent Parkway
Columbia, MD 21044-3263
Telephone: (410) 997–4040
E-mail: info@adta.org
Website: http://www.adta.org

This organization of dance therapists and practitioners acts as an information center, conducts workshops, and develops guidelines for educational and therapeutic programs.

American Massage Therapy Association (AMTA)
820 Davis Street, Suite 100
Evanston, IL 60201-4444
Telephone: (847) 864–0123

This nationwide organization provides information about massage therapy and furnishes referrals to local chapters.

American Occupational Therapy Association (AOTA)
4720 Montgomery Lane
P.O. Box 31220
Bethesda, MD 20824-1220
Telephone: (301) 652–2682
E-mail: practice@aota.org
Website: http://www.aota.org

This association offers a members' directory as well as advice and information about occupational therapy.

American Physical Therapy Association (APTA)
1111 North Fairfax Street
Alexandria, VA 22314
Telephone: (800) 999–2782
Website: http://www.apta.org

This organization seeks to educate the public about physical therapy and offers publications and referrals to local therapists.

American Polarity Therapy Association
2888 Bluff Street, Suite 149
Boulder, CO 80301
Telephone: (303) 545–2080
Website: http://userww.service.emory.edu/~labst/polarity/

This organization provides training, certification, and referrals to therapists in your locality.

American Society of Clinical Hypnosis (ASCH)
2200 East Devon Avenue, Suite 291
Des Plaines, IL 60018
Telephone: (847) 297–3317
Website: http://www.asch.net

This professional society provides educational material and is a referral source for local therapists. For information, please send a self-addressed stamped envelope.

Association for Applied Psychophysiology and Biofeedback
10200 West 44th Avenue, Suite 304
Wheat Ridge, CO 80033-2840

Telephone: (303) 422–8436
Fax: (303) 422–8894
E-mail: aapb@resourcenter.com
Website: http://www.aapb.org

This professional organization provides scientific and educational material. It is a referral source for local psychophysiologists.

Biofeedback Certification Institute of America
10200 West 44th Avenue, Suite 304
Wheat Ridge, CO 80033
Telephone: (303) 420–2902
E-mail: bcia@resourcenter.com

This institute can direct you to biofeedback practitioners in your area.

The Burdenko Institute
Water and Sports Therapy
475 Bedford Street
Lexington, MA 02173
Telephone: (617) 862–3727

The institute provides treatment and referrals for the Burdenko method. Igor Burdenko, Ph.D., director of the institute and creator of the Burdenko method, welcomes your questions.

California Yoga Teachers' Association (CYTA)
c/o Murria Frick Insurance
380 Stephens Avenue, First Floor
Solana Beach, CA 92075
Telephone: (800) 395–8075
Fax: (619) 259–6069

This association provides educational material and referrals for yoga therapists.

Center for Assistive Technology (CAT)
3100 Main Street
Kansas City, MO 64111
Telephone: (816) 931–2121

The center provides information and services to individuals with disabilities and their families and friends. Their computer program lists more than 20,000 assistive devices that help individuals with physical limitations. There is also a referral source to help people locate centers in specific localities.

Center for Coping
120 Bethpage Road, Suite 310
Hicksville, NY 11801
Telephone: (516) 822–3131
E-mail: Drbalance@aol.com

This multiservice organization helps individuals and family members improve their ability to deal with chronic medical problems through counseling.

Commission for Accreditation of Rehabilitation Facilities (CARF)
4891 East Grant Road
Tucson, AZ 85712
Telephone: (520) 325–1044
Fax: (520) 318–1129
Website: http://www.carf.org

This agency provides information about the accreditation of rehabilitation facilities and provides referrals for pain-management centers.

Feldenkrais Guild
P.O. Box 489
Albany, OR 97321
Telephone: (541) 926–0981
E-mail: feldngld@peak.org
Website: http://www.healthy.net/feldenkrais/

This association of certified practitioners and students strives to improve motor functioning and control related pain through education and retraining faulty movement patterns.

Jorge A. Gonzalez, M.D., Co-Medical Director
HealthSouth Rehab at Tulsa
3219 South 79 East Avenue
Tulsa, OK 74145
E-mail: jgrehab@aol.com
Website: rehabusa.com

Dr. Gonzalez is a neurologist with a specialty in neurorehabilitation and is the codirector of the Oklahoma Rehabilitation Hospital. He welcomes your questions.

HealthSouth Rehabilitation Institute of San Antonio (RIOSA)
9119 Cinnamon Hill
San Antonio, TX 78240
Telephone: (210) 691–0737
Website: http://www.healthsouth.com

This institute provides extensive rehabilitation services and furnishes literature and educational information to people in need of such assistance.

Herb Research Foundation
1007 Pearl Street, Suite 200
Boulder, CO 80302
Telephone: (303) 449–2265
E-mail: info@herbs.org
Website: http://www.herbs.org

This nonprofit research and educational organization collects and provides scientific and lay information about the use of herbs for health.

Homeopathic Educational Services
2124 Kittredge Street
Berkeley, CA 94704
Telephone: (510) 649–0294
E-mail: mail@homeopathic.com
Website: http://www.homeopathic.com

This organization provides access to a comprehensive assortment of homeopathic information, educational information, and products, as well as a directory of practitioners.

April Mott, M.D.
Taste and Smell Center
University of Connecticut Health Center
Farmington, CT 06030-5350
Telephone: (860) 679–2000
E-mail: amot@neuron.uchc.edu

Dr. Mott is the director of the chemosensory center. She welcomes your questions.

National Center for Homeopathy
801 North Fairfax Street, Suite 306
Alexandria, VA 22314
Telephone: (703) 548–7790
E-mail: nchinfo@igc.apc.org
Website: http://www.homeopathic.org

This organization provides educational information about homeopathic treatment and publishes a national directory of homeopaths.

National Commission for the Certification of Acupuncturists
P.O. Box 97075
Washington, DC 20090-7075
Telephone: (202) 232–1404
E-mail: ncca@compuserve.com

This nonprofit organization offers a national certification examination and can provide a list of certified acupuncturists.

National Easter Seal Society, Inc.
2030 West Monroe Street, Suite 1800
Chicago, IL 60606-4802
Telephone: (312) 726–6200, (800) 221–6827
TTY: (312) 726–4259
Website: http://www.seals.com

This organization provides direct rehabilitation services.

National Rehabilitation Information Center
8455 Colesville Road, Suite 935
Silver Spring, MD 20910
Telephone: (800) 346–2742
TTY: (301) 495–5626
Website: http://www.naric.com/naric

This agency provides audiovisual information on disabilities and rehabilitation and offers referrals to appropriate experts, programs, and facilities.

The Orton Dyslexia Society
Chester Building, Suite 382
8600 LaSalle Road
Baltimore, MD 21286-2044
Telephone: (410) 296–0232, (800) 222–3123
Fax: (410) 321–5069
Website: http://www.ods.org

This nonprofit organization exists to assist dyslexic children and adults through advocacy, research, education, and the promotion of specialized teaching approaches for people with learning disabilities. The society also provides referral lists of tutors within your locality.

The Society of Clinical and Experimental Hypnosis (SCEH)
3905 Vincennes Road, Suite 304
Indianapolis, IN 46268
Telephone: (317) 228–8073

Fax: (317) 872–7133
E-mail: lsshaw@aol.com
Website: http://www.spartan.ac.BrockU.CA/~wwwsceh/

This is a scientific and professional society for research on hypnosis. It provides referrals for therapists who do clinical hypnosis.

DISABILITY ISSUES

ADA Information Line
(202) 514–0301

This information service answers questions on requirements set forth by the Americans With Disabilities Act (ADA) and offers referrals to other government agencies involved with disability issues.

President's Committee on Employment of People With Disabilities
1331 F Street NW, Suite 300
Washington, DC 20004-1107
Telephone: (202) 376–6200
TTY: (202) 376–6205
Website: http://www.pcepd.gov

This agency works with a governor's committee for each state to advocate for employment and training opportunities for disabled people. The committee publishes the Directory of Organizations Interested in People With Disabilities.

FINANCIAL/INSURANCE CONCERNS

Insurance Information Institute
110 William Street
New York, NY 10038
Telephone: (800) 331–9146
Website: http://www.iii.org

This organization dispenses literature and information concerning homeowner's and automobile insurance.

National Consumers League
1701 K Street NW, Suite 1200
Washington, DC 20006
Telephone: (202) 835–3323
E-mail: nclncl@aol.com

This organization conducts research and sponsors educational and advocacy programs on such consumer issues as insurance, credit, health, and privacy.

National Foundation for Consumer Credit
8611 Second Avenue, Suite 100
Silver Spring, MD 20910
Telephone: (800) 388-2227 (touch-tone), (301) 589-5600 (rotary)

This agency provides referrals to local nonprofit credit-counseling agencies.

National Insurance Consumer Helpline
Telephone: (800) 942–4242

This nationwide hotline provides assistance and answers to persons with problems and questions related to insurance coverage.

REHABILITATION AND ASSISTIVE PRODUCTS AND TECHNOLOGY

ABLEDATA System
8455 Colesville Road, Suite 935
Silver Spring, MD 20910
Telephone: (800) 227–0216
Website: http://www.abledata.com

This organization provides information about assistive technology. In maintains a database on some 23,000 items. It is also a referral source for assistive technology for specific daily living activities.

Books on Tape
P.O. Box 7900
Newport Beach, CA 92660
Telephone: (800) 252–6996
Fax: (714) 548–6574
Website: http://www.booksontape.com

This company offers audiotaped versions of classic and popular books.

Creative Labs, Inc.
Creative Labs Customer Service
P.O. Box 1452
Stillwater, OK 74076
Telephone: (800) 998–1000
Website: http://www.creativelabs.com

This corporation makes Soundblaster sound cards for computers. Text Assist, a Windows-based software product that is included with most Soundblaster sound cards, will read aloud what is on a computer screen.

Crestwood Company
6625 North Sidney Place
Milwaukee, WI 53209-3259
Telephone: (414) 352–5678
Helpline: (414) 352–HELP (ask to speak with Ruth Leff, Speech/ Language Pathologist)
Fax: (414) 352–5679
E-mail: Crestcomm@aol.com
Website: http://www.communicationaids.com

This company provides easy-to-use communication aids for children and adults, including over 275 high-tech and low-tech devices. Free catalogue available.

Evelyn Wood Reading Dynamics
Telephone: (800) 447–7323

Offers reading programs that may be helpful to some people recovering from MTBI.

HumanWare Inc.
6245 King Road
Loomis, CA 95650
Telephone: (800) 722–3393
E-mail: info@humanware.com
Website: http://www.humanware.com

This corporation makes Soundproof, a PC device that provides a small voice synthesizer and a tracking system that lets you hear what appears on a computer monitor rather than having to read it.

The Learning Company
1 Athenaeum Street
Cambridge, MA 02142
Telephone: (800) 227–5609
Website: http://www.learningco.com

This company offers a of software, games, and other teaching aids for adults and children. Free catalogue available.

Nightingale/Conant
7300 North Lehigh
Niles, IL 60714
Telephone: (800) 323–5552
Website: http://www.nightgale.com

This company manufactures Kevin Trudeau's Mega Memory, a series of audiotapes that teach easy-to-learn memory techniques. The company also offers audiotapes to improve self-esteem and facilitate relaxation.

Sportime International
1 Sportime Way
Atlanta, GA 30340
Telephone: (800) 444–5700
E-mail: orders@sportime.com; catalog.request@sportime.com

This company offers specialized rehabilitative equipment for fun and move-ment. It puts out several different types of catalogues: Abilitations (equipment for development and restoration of physical and mental ability through move-ment) and Chime Time (for preschool, elementary, and special populations).

Xerox Imaging System, Inc.
9 Centennial Drive
Peabody, MA 01960
Telephone: (508) 977–2000, (800) 248–6550
Fax: (508) 977–2148
Website: http://www.xerox.com

This company has developed Bookwise, a PC-based interactive system for in-dividuals with learning disabilities or TBI. The system scans books and other printed materials, converts the text to synthesized speech, and highlights text by word, phrase, sentence, or line, thus providing visual and audio tracking assistance.

OTHER

Kenneth I. Kolpan, Esq.
Law Office of Kenneth I. Kolpan, P.C.
100 Summer Street, Suite 3232
Boston, MA 02110
Telephone: (617) 426–2558

Mr. Kolpan is the author of numerous articles on legal issues related to TBI and a member of editorial board for The Journal of Head Trauma Reha-bilitation.

National Organization for Victim Assistance (NOVA)
1757 Park Road, NW
Washington, DC 20010
Telephone: (202) 232–6682
E-mail: nova@access.digex.net
Website: http://www.access.digex.net/~nova

This agency works to express victims' claims for decency, compassion, and jus-tice. NOVA wishes to ensure that victims' rights are honored by government officials and others who can aid in recovery.

National Victim Center
2111 Wilson Boulevard, Suite 300
Arlington, VA 22201
Telephone: (703) 276–2880
E-mail: nvc@mail.org.nvc
Website: http://www.nvc.org

The center's goal is to function as a national resource center to seek redress for injustices done to crime victims. National referrals and educational information are offered.

Outdoor Camping
Camp Hemlocks
Massachusetts Brain Association
484 Main Street, Suite 325
Worcester, MA 01608
Telephone: (508) 795–0244, (800) 242–0030

This camp for adults ages sixteen to forty-five with TBI is designed to promote independence and provide summer fun.

Charles N. Simkins, Esq.
Simkins & Simkins, P.C.
Attorneys at Law
200 North Center Street
Northville, MI 48167-1416
Telephone: (810) 349–6030
E-mail: SimkinsR@aol.com

Mr. Simkins is the author of a series of thirteen essays on legal issues regarding TBI.

INDIVIDUAL CONTACTS

Diane Roberts Stoler, Ed.D.
P.O. Box 148
Georgetown, MA 01833
Telephone: (978) 352–6349
E-mail: dianes@shore.net, dianes@mediaone.net
On-line E-mail: Dianes5119 (AOL) VPGC96A (Prodigy)

If you are interested in making individual contacts with other brain-injured people, please write to me.

REFERENCES FOR FURTHER READING

Listed below are books, periodicals, and other publications addressing different aspects of MTBIs and their treatment. These can be valuable sources of information for the person who has suffered a brain injury as well as for his or her loved ones.

BRAIN INJURY—GENERAL

Bryant, Beverley. *In Search of Wings.* South Paris, ME: Wing Publications, 1992.

——*To Wherever Oceans Go.* South Paris, ME: Wing Publications, 1996.

Campbell, Kay, and Constance Miller. *From The Ashes: A Head Injury Self-Advocacy Guide.* Seattle, WA: The Phoenix Project, 1987.

DeBoskey, Dana S., Ph.D., and Connie J. Calub, M.D. *Life After Head Injury: Who Am I?* Houston, TX: HDI Publishers, 1989.

Eutsey, Dwayne E. *Brain Injury—Survivor and Caregiver Education Manual.* Gaithersburg, MD: Aspen Publications Inc., 1996.

Felton, Patricia, Ed. *Through This Window: Views on Traumatic Brain Injury.* Brooks, ME: EBTS, Inc., 1992.

Head Injury Update. HDI Publishers, P.O. Box 131401, Houston, TX 77219.

Lehmkuhl, Don, Ph.D., Ed. *Brain Injury Glossary.* Houston, TX: HDI Publishers, 1992.

Mercer, Dorothy L., Ph.D. *Injury: Learning to Live Again.* Ventura, CA: Pathfinders Publishing, 1994.

TPN Magazine. The Perspectives Network, P.O. Box 1859, Cumming, GA 30128.

Pflug, Jackie Nink. *Miles To Go Before I Sleep.* Center City, MN: Hazelden, 1996.

Rizzo, Matthew, and Daniel Tranel, Eds. *Head Injury and Post Concussive Syndrome.* New York, NY: Churchill Livingston, 1996.

Saperstein, Robert, J.D., and Dana Saperstein, Ph.D. *Surviving an Auto Accident: A Guide to Your Physical, Economic, and Emotional Recovery.* Ventura, CA: Pathfinders Publishing, 1994.

Swiercinsky, Dennis P., Ph.D., Terrie L. Price, Ph.D., and Leif Eric Leaf, Ph.D. *Traumatic Head Injury: Causes, Consequence, and Challenge.* Kansas City, MO: The Head Injury Association of Kansas and Greater Kansas City, Inc, 1993.

Whitman, Ruth A. *Making Sense Out of Nonsense: Models of Head Injury Rehabilitation.* Ontario, Canada: Rehab Publishing, 1994.

PHYSICAL SYMPTOMS

American Council on Headache Education, with Lynne M. Constantine and Suzanne Scott. *Migraine: The Complete Guide.* New York, NY: Dell, 1994.

Bell, David S., M.D., and Stef Donev. *Curing Fatigue: A Step-by-Step Plan to Uncover and Eliminate the Causes of Chronic Fatigue.* Emmaus, PA: Rodale Press, 1993.

Bergman, Thomas. *Moments That Disappear: Children Living With Epilepsy.* Milwaukee, WI: Gareth Stevens Publishers, 1992.

Buchan, Neil. *Epilepsy and You: Information For People With Epilepsy, Parents, Teachers, and Other Interested Persons.* Baltimore, MD: Williams and Wilkins Associates, 1987.

Cauldill, Margaret A., M.D., Ph.D. *Managing Pain Before It Manages You.* New York, NY: Guilford Press, 1995.

Combs, Alec. *Hearing Loss Help*. San Luis Obispo, CA: Impact Publishers, 1991.

Consumer Reports Book Editors. *Hearing Loss Handbook*. Yonkers, NY: Consumer Reports Books, 1993.

Corey, David, and Stan Solomon. *Pain: Free Yourself for Life*. New York, NY: NAL-Dutton, 1989.

D'Alonzo, T.L., O.D. *Your Eyes: A Comprehensive Look at the Understanding and Treatment of Vision Problems*. Clifton Heights, PA: Avanti Publishing, 1991.

Donoghue, Paul J., Ph.D., and Mary E. Siegel, Ph.D. *Sick and Tired of Feeling Sick and Tired: Living With Invisible Chronic Illness*. New York, NY: W.W. Norton & Co., 1992.

Freeman, John M., M.D., Eileen Vining, P.G., and Diana Pillas. *Seizures and Epilepsy in Childhood: A Guide for Parents*. Baltimore, MD: The Johns Hopkins University Press, 1990.

Griffith, Ernest R., and Sally Lemberg. *Sexuality and the Person With Traumatic Brain Injury—A Guide for Families*. Philadelphia, PA: F.A. Davis Co., 1993.

Headley, Barbara J. *Chronic Pain: Life Out of Balance*. St. Paul, MN: Pain Resources Limited, 1988.

Landau, Elaine. *Epilepsy*. New York, NY: Twenty-First Century Books, 1994.

LaPlante, Eve. *Seized*. New York, NY: HarperCollins, 1991.

McIlwain, Harris H., M.D., Bruce and Debra Fulgham, and Joel C. Silverfield, M.D. *Winning With Back Pain*. New York, NY: John Wiley & Sons, 1994.

Mohr-Catalano, Ellen M., Ed. *Chronic Pain Control Work Book*. Oakland, CA: New Harbinger, 1987.

People's Medical Society. *Options in Health Care: Understanding Traditional and Alternative Methods*. Allentown, PA: People's Medical Society, 1985.

Rapoport, Alan, M.D., and Fred D. Sheftell, M.D. *Headache Relief.* New York, NY: Fireside Books, 1991.

Rosenfeld, Isadore, M.D. *Symptoms.* New York, NY: Bantam Books, 1989.

Sachellares, J. Chris, and Stanley Berent. *Psychological Disturbances in Epilepsy.* Boston, MA: Butterworth-Heinemann, 1996.

Saper, Joel R. *Help for Headaches: A Guide to Understanding Their Causes and Finding the Best Methods of Treatment.* New York, NY: Warner Books, 1987.

Schachter, Steven C., Ed. *Brainstorms—Epilepsy in Our Words: Personal Accounts of Living With Seizures.* New York, NY: Raven Press, 1993.

Solomon, Seymour, M.D., and Steven Fraccaro. *The Headache Book: Effective Treatments to Prevent Headaches and Relieve Pain.* Mt. Vernon, NY: Consumer Reports Books, 1991.

Spierings, Egilius, L.H. *Management of Migraine.* Boston, MA: Butterworth-Heinemann, 1996.

Stacy, Charles B., Andrew S. Kaplan, and Gray Williams. *The Fight Against Pain.* Yonkers, NY: Consumer Reports Books, 1992.

Sternbach, Richard A. *Mastering Pain: A Twelve-Step Program for Coping with Chronic Pain.* New York, NY: Putnam, 1987.

COGNITIVE SYMPTOMS

Clayton, Lawrence, and Jaydene Morrison. *Coping With a Learning Disability.* New York, NY: Rosen Publishing Group, 1992.

Cummings, Rhoda Woods, and Gary L. Fisher. *The School Survival Guide For Kids With LD* (*learning differences).* Minneapolis, MN: Free Spirit Publications, 1991.

Downing, David. *303 Dumb Spelling Misstakes and What You Can Do About Them.* Lincolnwood, IL: National Textbook Co., 1990.

Fogler, Janet. *Improving Your Memory: How To Remember What You're Starting to Forget.* Baltimore, MD: Johns Hopkins University Press, 1994.

Fry, Ronald W. *Improve Your Memory.* Hawthorne, NJ: Career Press, 1994.

Hayes, Marnell L. *You Don't Outgrow It: Living With Learning Disabilities.* Novato, CA: Academic Therapy Publications, 1993.

Hartmann, Thom. *Attention Deficit Disorder: A Different Perception.* Grass Valley, CA: Underwood Books, 1993.

Horn, Sam. *Concentration! How to Focus for Success.* Menlo Park, CA: Crisp Publications, 1991.

Kelly, Kate. *You Mean I'm Not Lazy, Stupid, or Crazy? A Self-Help Book For Adults With Attention Deficit Disorder.* New York, NY: Scribner, 1995.

Leviton, Richard. *Brain Builders!* West Nyack, NY: Parker Publishing Co., 1995.

Moss, Robert A. *Why Johnny Can't Concentrate: Coping With Attention Deficit Problems.* New York, NY: Bantam, 1990.

Murphy, Kevin R. *Out of the Fog: Treatment Options and Coping Strategies for Adult Attention Deficit Disorder.* Westport, CT: Hyperion, 1995.

Mark, Vernon H. *Reversing Memory Loss: Proven Methods for Regaining, Strengthening, and Preserving Your Memory.* Boston, MA: Houghton-Mifflin, 1992.

Parker, Rolland S., Ph.D. *Traumatic Brain Injury and Neuropsychological Impairment.* New York, NY: Springer-Verlag, 1990.

Peterson, Harold A., and Thomas P. Marquardt. *Appraisal and Diagnosis of Speech and Language Disorders.* New York: Prentice Hall, 1990.

Ruchlis, Hyman. *Clear Thinking: A Practical Introduction.* Buffalo, NY: Prometheus, 1990.

Selikowitz, Mark. *Dyslexia and Other Learning Difficulties: The Facts.* New York, NY: Oxford University Press, 1992.

Sullivan, George. *Work Smart, Not Hard.* New York, NY: Facts on File, 1987.

Winston, Stephanie. *Stephanie Winston's Best Organizing Tips: Quick, Simple Ways to Get Organized and Get On With Your Life.* New York, NY: Simon and Schuster, 1995.

PSYCHOLOGICAL SYMPTOMS

Buckingham, Robert W. *Coping With Grief.* New York: Rosen Publishing Group, 1991.

Casarijan, Robin. *Forgiveness: A Bold Choice for a Peaceful Heart.* New York, NY: Bantam Books, 1992.

Colgrove, Melba, Ph.D., Harold H. Bloomfield, M.D., and Peter McWilliams. *How to Survive the Loss of a Love: 58 Things To Do When There Is Nothing To Be Done.* New York, NY: Bantam Books, 1981.

Hales, Diane R. *Caring For the Mind: The Comprehensive Guide to Mental Health.* New York: Bantam Books, 1994.

Heston, Leonard L. *Mending Minds: A Guide to the New Psychiatry of Depression, Anxiety, and Other Mental Disorders.* New York: W.H. Freeman, 1992.

Howard, Michael, and Joseph Bleiberg. *A Manual of Behavior Management Strategies for Traumatically Brain Injured Adults.* Chicago, IL: Rehabilitation Institute of Chicago, 1982.

Rank, Maureen. *Free to Grieve.* Minneapolis, MN: Bethany House, 1985.

Singer, Lilly. *Beyond Loss: A Practical Guide Through Grief to a Meaningful Life.* New York: Dutton, 1988.

Verninga, Robert L. *A Gift of Hope.* Boston: Little, Brown, and Co., 1985.

FAMILY ISSUES

Anderson, Janet, Ph.D., and Frederick Parente. "Training Family Members to Work With the Head Injured Patient." Article available through the Brain Injury Association, 1776 Massachusetts Avenue NW, Suite 100, Washington, DC 20036-1904.

Barry, Philip, Ph.D. "Family Adjustment to Head Injury." Article available through the Brain Injury Association of Kansas and Greater Kansas City, 110 Pennsylvania Avenue, Suite 4061, Kansas City, MO 64105-1356.

"Helpful Suggestions in Relating to Your Family Member With Head Injury." Article available through the Brain Injury Association of Kansas and Greater Kansas City, 110 Pennsylvania Avenue, Suite 4061, Kansas City, MO 64105-1356.

Hutchison, Ruth, M.S. and Terry Hutchison, M.D., Ph.D. *Head Injury: A Booklet for Families.* Houston: Texas Brain Injury Foundation, 1983.

Hutzler, Cynthia. "The Head Injured Child: Loss, Grief, and Sorrow." Article available through the Brain Injury Association of Kansas and Greater Kansas City, 110 Pennsylvania Avenue, Suite 4061, Kansas City, MO 64105-1356.

Lash, Marilyn, M.S.W. "When a Parent Has a Brain Injury: Sons and Daughters Speak Out." Article available through the New Hampshire Brain Injury Association, 2½ Beacon Street, Concord, NH 03301-4447.

———"When Your Child Goes to School After an Injury." Article available through the Brain Injury Association, 1776 Massachusetts Avenue NW, Suite 100, Washington, DC 20036-1904.

———"When Your Child Is Seriously Injured: The Emotional Impact on Families." Article available through the Brain Injury Association, 1776 Massachusetts Avenue NW, Suite 100, Washington, DC 20036-1904.

Leaf, Leif E., Ph.D. "Susan's Dad: A Child's Story of Head Injury." Article available through the Brain Injury Association, 1776 Massachusetts Avenue NW, Suite 100, Washington, DC 20036-1904.

Lezak, Muriel D. "Brain Damage is a Family Affair." Article available through the Brain Injury Association, 1776 Massachusetts Avenue NW, Suite 100, Washington, DC 20036-1904.

———"Psychological Implication of Traumatic Brain Damage for the Patient's Family." Article available through the Brain Injury Association, 1776 Massachusetts Avenue NW, Suite 100, Washington, DC 20036-1904.

Senelick, Richard C., M.D., and Cathy E. Ryan. *Living With Head Injury: A Guide for Families.* Washington, DC: Rehabilitation Hospital Services Corporation, 1991.

William, Janet M., and Thomas Kay, Eds. *Head Injury: A Family Matter.* Baltimore, MD: Paul H. Brooks Publishing Co., 1991.

Zeigler, Elizabeth. "Spouses of Persons Who Are Brain Injured: Overlooked Victims." Article available through the Brain Injury Association of Kansas and Greater Kansas City, 1100 Pennsylvania Avenue, Suite 4061, Kansas City, MO 64105-1356.

LEGAL AND INSURANCE ISSUES

Inlander, Charles R., and Charles K. Mackay. *Medicare Made Easy.* Reading, MA: Addison-Wesley, 1992.

Lunt, Suzanne. *A Handbook for the Disabled.* New York, NY: Charles Scribner's Sons, 1982.

TREATMENT APPROACHES

Adamovich, Brenda, Jennifer Henderson, and Sanford Auerbach. *Cognitive Rehabilitation of Closed Head Injured Patients.* Austin, TX: College-Hill Press, 1985.

Bach Flower Essences for the Family. London, England: Wigmore, 1993.

Benson, Herbert. *The Relaxation Response.* New York, NY: Avon, 1976.

Bengali, Vivian, Ed. *Head Injury in Children and Adolescents: A Resource and Review Book for School and Allied Professionals.* Brandon, VT: Clinical Psychology Publishing Co., Inc., 1992.

Brubaker, S.H. *Workbook for Reasoning Skill: Exercises for Cognitive Facilitation.* Detroit, MI: Wayne State University Press, 1985.

Burke, William, Ph.D. *Head Injury Rehabilitation: An Overview.* Houston, TX: HDI Publishers, 1989.

Calub, Connie, and Dana S. Deboskey. *Head Injury: A Home Based Cognitive Rehabilitation Program.* Houston, TX: HDI Publishers, 1989.

Goleman, Daniel, Ph.D., and Joel Gurin. *Mind/Body Medicine: How To Use Your Mind for Better Health.* Yonkers, NY: Consumer Reports Books, 1993.

Hallowell, Michael. *Herbal Healing: A Practical Introduction to Medicinal Herbs.* Garden City Park, NY: Avery Publishing Group, 1994.

Journal of Cognitive Rehabilitation (bimonthly magazine). 6555 Carollton Avenue, Indianapolis, IN 46220.

Kreutzer, Jeffrey, M.D. *Cognitive Rehabilitation for Persons With Traumatic Brain Injury: A Functional Approach.* Baltimore, MD: Paul H. Brooks, 1991.

Krupp, Marcus, and Milton L. Chatton. *Current Medical Diagnosis and Treatment.* Los Altos, CA: Appleton-Lange, 1987.

Lieberman, Shari, and Nancy Bruning. *The Real Vitamin & Mineral Book: Going Beyond the RDA for Optimum Health.* Garden City Park, NY: Avery Publishing Group, 1997.

Pinckney, Cathey, and Edward R. Pinckney. *The Patient's Guide to Medical Tests.* New York, NY: Facts on File, 1987.

Smith, Dorothy L. *Medication Guide for Patient Counseling.* Philadelphia, PA: Lea and Febiger, 1981.

Sobel, David S., M.D., and Tom Ferguson, M.D. *People's Book of Medical Tests.* New York, NY: Summit Books, 1984.

Stein, Diane. *The Natural Remedy Book for Women.* Freedom, CA: The Crossing Press, 1992.

Weiner, Michael. *The Complete Book of Homeopathy.* Garden City Park, NY: Avery Publishing Group, 1989.

Wigmore, Ann. *Why Suffer? How I Overcame Illness & Pain Naturally.* Garden City Park, NY: Avery Publishing Group, 1985.

Wilson, Roberta. *Aromatherapy for Vibrant Health and Beauty.* Garden City Park, NY: Avery Publishing Group, 1995.

Yoga Journal. Goodfellow Publishers, 2054 University Avenue, Suite 501, Berkeley, CA 94704.

OTHER

Jaffee, Kenneth M., and Ross M. Hays. *Pediatric Head Injury Rehabilitative Medical Management.* Brain Injury Association, 1776 Massachusetts Avenue NW, Suite 100, Washington, DC 20036-1904.

Moving Forward (monthly newspaper). P.O. Box 3553, Torrance, CA 90510-3553.

Warrington, Janette. *The Humpty Dumpty Syndrome.* Winona Lake, IN: Light and Life Press, 1991.

INDEX

Page numbers followed by (f) indicate figures. Those followed by (t) indicate tables.